'I WISH I'D KNOWN EARLIER ...'

MENOPAUSE: SURVIVE AND THRIVE

Anne Hope

BSc (Hons) PGCE LCCH RSHom

Claire Chaubert

BSc (Hons) LCCH RSHom RM

First published in 2017 by Telos Publishing Ltd,

5A Church Road, Shortlands, Bromley, Kent

BR2 0HP, United Kingdom.

www.telos.co.uk

Menopause: Survive and Thrive © 2017 Anne Hope
and Claire Chaubert

Design: Mark Stammers

ISBN: 978-1-84583-953-6

Disclaimer:

This book is for information and education purposes only. It is not intended to and does not offer individual medical advice or diagnosis to any reader. Telos Publishing Ltd accepts no responsibility or liability for the products, services or websites of any other companies mentioned in the text.

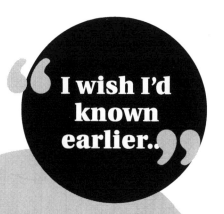

"I wish I'd known earlier.."

Menopause: Survive and Thrive

CONTENTS

AUTHORS' NOTE

The individual experiences recounted in this book are drawn from real clients we have seen in our clinic in South London. However, the names and potentially identifying details have been changed to protect their identities and confidentiality.

We love to have your feedback, so please feel free to get in touch with us via Twitter, Facebook or our website at www. naturalbornhealers.co.uk, where you can sign up for podcasts.

Anne Hope and Claire Chaubert

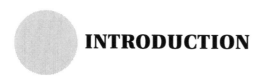

INTRODUCTION

This book has come about as a result of our work with many women who over the years have sought our advice and help on issues relating to the menopause. These woman have come to our clinic experiencing all manner of symptoms, both physical and emotional. As a result, we have developed a range of treatments and strategies that really work.

Whether you are simply looking ahead and wondering what the menopause might hold for you, or whether you are actually experiencing symptoms right now and don't know what to do next, this book is for you.

We give detailed explanations so that you can gain a better understanding of the processes that take place during menopause. It is quite surprising how much misinformation and negativity have been absorbed into women's consciousness over the years! We also go through the most common questions and problems that women bring to our clinic, and suggest lots of practical solutions and approaches.

More than this, we want to get the message out there: the menopause is an important and joyful journey. It allows us to enter a new phase of our life with awareness and become free to channel our energy into creativity and intellectual endeavour. It is a time of transition, and this means remaking the patterns of our life into a conscious and wonderful finale.

This book will enable you to develop your own personal action plan, and not just to survive but to thrive in and beyond the menopause.

The first chapter gives you lots of basic information about the menopause – use this as you want and return to it as a reference. The other chapters deal with the most common issues that women tell us are important to them, and that arise over and over. We also cover the joy of 'waking up' into this amazing time of creativity and freedom, exploring and finding our true nature.

Because we want this book to be useful as well as informative, we have set out at the end of each chapter some options for treatments that we have found to be helpful in alleviating women's symptoms. Then, at the end of the book, we have summarised some of the main options, for ease of reference.

By giving information about the common symptoms of menopause, and suggesting different ways of managing them, we aim to help you to find an approach that works best for you. The treatments we suggest are not the only ones that exist, but they are commonly available, and have been reliably shown to help women we have seen in our clinic. We urge you to ensure that you source the best quality supplements and remedies possible. Quality matters.

Suggested approaches to address particular symptoms or issues are grouped at the end of each chapter as follows:

Diet and vitamin supplements

Enhancing your diet with foods or supplements that contain particular vitamins or minerals will have a direct effect on the body. In times of major change, such as the menopause, the body can need different things than usual – so these are important. The quality of vitamins matters enormously. They should always be in a food state (also described as bioavailable) so that the body can absorb them correctly and avoid having to deal with synthetic copies, which can be of little or no benefit. The packaging will always indicate when vitamins are in a food state. Cheaper products are generally not in this form; the vitamins are synthetically produced from chemicals.

A possible downside of adjusting your diet is that it can impact on your individual lifestyle. If this is the case for you, perhaps making just one or two changes, or taking a few good-quality supplements along with other treatments, might be the best approach.

Herbal supplements

Herbal supplements will again have a direct effect on the body. It is worth remembering that just because something is described as natural, this doesn't mean it is safe to take lots of it – after all, snake venom is natural! Herbs are traditionally a very effective and common way of managing hormonal symptoms. In this book, we discuss various different individual herbs and their effects on the body. Although some manufacturers offer menopause preparations that consist of a mix of several herbs, we have taken the view that understanding the individual herbs that are most useful in the treatment of particular symptoms will help you to choose. The herbs contained in a mix will often be present in low amounts, and you might decide that you would actually benefit from having higher amounts of one or two of them. You might also prefer to avoid taking certain herbs if you feel you don't need those specific ones.

Again, how a herb is extracted is paramount to its efficacy. Quality matters. It doesn't always follow that the greater the amount of a herb, the greater its effect. The way it is extracted and manufactured has a direct effect on the way it is absorbed by the body.

We have successfully used a couple of trusted manufacturers, but would always advise you to shop around. In addition, because of the way herbs work, you should always consult your health professional to check on possible interactions with other medications.

Homeopathic remedies

Homeopathy is designed to have a balancing effect on the body, getting it to work at its best and thereby relieving adverse symptoms. This means that it works slightly differently from the above two approaches, which directly 'push' the body.

There are thousands of homeopathic remedies available, and differentiating between them and deciding on the best ones to suit you is not always easy. In this book we indicate the most common remedies shown to be broadly effective for particular symptoms. In the UK, there are three main homeopathic pharmacies that make remedies. They stock them all, and make them available to order online via their websites. A very limited selection is also available from some chemists and health shops. Whenever you take homeopathic remedies, you should always be careful to ensure that they are from a reliable source.

Australian Bush Flower Remedies

Australian Bush Flower Remedies are a set of fifty flower remedies that are carefully grown and harvested in such a way as to maintain their healing properties. They can be extremely helpful and wide-ranging in their effects, and are completely safe, so they can be a good starting point if you are looking for support. They are different from herbs, in that they are intended to be more holistic in their action. Although they are widely available, their manufacture is protected by trademarks, and this ensures their efficacy.

Bach Flower Remedies

Bach Flower Remedies are a set of 38 flowers – again protected in their growth and manufacture to ensure their integrity. They are widely available and safe, can be used repeatedly, and can provide excellent relief during acute situations. They can be a good choice if you prefer to begin with a very gentle approach.

Some other suggestions, tips and ideas have been included in each chapter to help you to find the right approach for you.

We cannot stress enough that taking control of this new phase of your life will lay the foundations for you to have a powerful and exciting future.

Happy reading and ageing!

1 UNDERSTANDING THE MENOPAUSE

The menopause is not well understood, and is often characterised as a grim process that all women have to endure. Consequently, quite reasonably, many women feel very concerned about it, or even dread it.

This book is a guide to how to survive and thrive in what is actually a new and exciting time in your life. It will give you the information you need to:

- understand the basics of what happens during the menopause, and why;

- learn more about common symptoms;

- realise that there are steps you can take to pass through the menopause with ease;

- think through all the options and choices you have;

- develop a practical and achievable action plan so that you are in charge of your life during your menopause; and

- help you truly embrace and welcome the power, freedom and opportunities that this new phase will bring you.

CASE STUDY – THERESA

'I was having hot flushes, which were annoying, and my sleep was affected. And as my periods were becoming on and off, I thought that meant I must be menopausal, and that I was running out of all my hormones. I was worried about my bones, and wondered what I needed to do. It was only then I realised how little I knew about what was really happening. It felt a bit frightening – which, when I look back, seems crazy, as this is a normal process for women.'

A lot of women who come to see us in our clinic are suffering symptoms of menopause. They are concerned about managing their general health now that this change has begun; about the risk of deterioration of their bones; and about how to cope with a general lack of energy. They often report feeling suddenly old. It seems a very commonly-held misconception that hormones all stop at this point, and everything then goes downhill. It can feel frightening, like a sudden loss. Our clients want to find a way to cope with all of this.

Actually, though, passing through the menopause should not be about coping with 'the awfulness of this time', nor about 'getting used to things being not as good as they were before' – both of which phrases we have often heard used. It is a time of transformation, yes, but not – as it is often portrayed – a time of deficiency, coping and loss. Instead, correctly, it should be a time of transformation into creativity, freedom and health. We help women to understand and live this, in a practical way.

'The change' ... !

How often have you heard young people say that they dread 'going into menopause'; or, worse, recount stories about their own mother or aunt turning into some kind of 'old dragon' one day and never being the same again? Small wonder so many women dread and fear this time. So often we think of it as the end of our being attractive or just of being ourselves as we know it.

Many women believe that because their bleed stops, they lose all their oestrogen, and that with no hormones circulating anymore, their symptoms are inevitable; so any bodily changes simply have to be accepted and got used to. This is not true.

In years gone by, when women talked to each other about the menopause, the expression they often used (or probably mouthed, if children were present) was 'the change'. This is actually not a bad description, as the menopause is in fact a transition. It is not the end of hormones, but a change in where the body manufactures them and how it uses them.

This is a natural process that you can positively influence by taking some important steps, which we will be describing in subsequent chapters. Hormones have an enormous emotional impact as well as a physiological one. Managing the changes that take place is a path to power and wisdom, and potentially feeling the fittest and freest you have ever felt.

In short, struggling for years against the tide of symptoms is not necessary; becoming a dragon and the dread of your family is not inevitable. The menopause can actually be your path to empowerment, allowing you to make the most of the precious later years of your life; and we have helped many women to discover this secret.

CASE STUDY – CAROLINE

Caroline came to see us. She was 59 and had been suffering hot flushes and mood-swings. At night her flushes were so severe that she had to keep towels in the bed, regularly changing them as they got wet from her sweating so much. She was up two or three times a night to change her nightclothes and the towels. She couldn't share the bed with her partner anymore. During the day she was exhausted, and at work had to keep hiding from clients as the flushes made her red-faced, hot and sweaty. She also felt anxious for no reason – and she hadn't been this way before. She wondered how long her husband would put up with her down moods. She didn't want to go out anymore, or see friends as she had done in the past. To make things worse, she had been suffering like this for over 13 years, constantly being told that it might last just another couple of years and then get better. She didn't feel it was getting better. In fact, over the last few months things had got worse. Her husband had said she needed to do something for both their sakes.

Caroline is quite typical of the women we see in our clinic. They wait until life becomes almost beyond rescue before desperately looking for some assistance. We were actually able to help Caroline at her first appointment. Possibly because her body was so ready to pass through and find balance, once it got a nudge in the right direction, it continued to right itself very quickly. But the main point here is how many women expect to have severe, life-disrupting symptoms. No wonder it is the 'dreaded' menopause! We want to spread the word that it doesn't have to be that way.

In this first chapter, we will explain the basics of what actually happens to our bodies during the menopause, and why.

Menopause – the process

Strictly speaking, 'menopause ' means the final period that a woman has; the word derives from Greek, in which 'meno' means month and 'pausis' means stop. However, 'menopause' is commonly used to describe the whole phase a woman goes through, often for some years before and after the last menstruation.

The correct word to describe the whole transition is actually 'climacteric'. This encompasses the time from the very beginning of the change in female hormones, through the common symptoms of irregular menstrual cycles, to the ending of menstrual bleed, after which the hormones settle into a new natural pattern. During this time, the production of oestrogen and progesterone slows down as the body changes from an age of child-bearing capability to past child-bearing capability. As a result of these changes, women can experience physical symptoms such as:

- irregular periods, which can range from very heavy or even flooding to a light, non-stop flow; to a dark, sluggish bleed; or to an erratic light bleed;

- hot flushes, or hot flashes, which can be short and sharp or can last longer, causing disruptive sweating;

- inability to control internal temperature, so that once the body starts becoming hot or cold it just seems to continue;

- alterations in sleep patterns, flushes disrupting sleep, and difficulty in falling or staying asleep;

- changes in libido, and vaginal dryness;

- mood-swings, low mood, weepiness, irritability, tearfulness, or just a down or flat feeling, often for no real reason;

- anxiety, or inability to do things – such as driving, or giving a presentation at work – that previously could be achieved with confidence;

- memory loss, or a strange disconnected feeling, not always feeling in touch with what is happening;

- feeling at the end of useful life, or even experiencing depression.

Sounds really worrying – no wonder that our case study client Theresa felt apprehensive!

Many women find themselves unprepared for these symptoms. This is similar to the situation where, in years gone by, girls would often begin their periods in terror, as no-one had prepared them for the onset of puberty. Luckily we have moved forward from that, and now prepare girls (and hopefully boys too) with information about exactly what will happen, and why, and what symptoms they (or their girlfriends) are likely to be having. However, it is our observation that many women still learn about their menopause only as they live through it; and men are largely ignorant about what their partners are experiencing.

We always tell our clients that menopause is a time of transition and not 'the end' of their hormones. Beforehand, they will have lived for many years with their hormones being produced and running a certain way, with monthly cycles of oestrogen and progesterone. This has become characteristic, and formed part of who they are. But with the onset of menopause, they do not simply have to 'go without'. It is really just a reorganisation of how the body works. Too often it is considered a pathological condition for which medical intervention is needed, when actually it is a completely natural process.

The technical bit ...

So, let's look at the science behind the process.

There are two hormones that are most influential throughout a woman's life, and these are oestrogen and progesterone. They come in strongly at puberty, starting the menstrual cycle and the big emotional changes that accompany the transition from a girl into a woman, and all the complexities that brings.

At puberty, a part of the brain called the hypothalamus is triggered to secrete a hormone that stimulates the pituitary gland. This in turn stimulates the ovaries to produce oestrogen and progesterone. Although it isn't known exactly why this occurs when it does, it seems to coincide with when body fat reaches a level of about 17%-20% of body weight. Girls over 16 need a minimum ratio of 22% body fat to body weight in order to maintain a regular menstrual cycle.[1] Studies suggest that this figure is critical, indicating that a particular body fat ratio is needed to establish and maintain a healthy hormonal balance.

These two main hormones of oestrogen and progesterone run the menstrual cycle. Oestrogen is dominant in the first half of the cycle, rising until ovulation occurs, when it drops away. Progesterone then builds in the second half of the cycle, after ovulation, preparing the body for potential pregnancy. At the end of the cycle, if there is no fertilised egg, the progesterone level drops and a bleed occurs; if there is a fertilised egg, meaning that the woman is pregnant, the progesterone level continues to rise.

Assuming that a woman is not having any form of chemical contraception (i.e. the contraceptive pill, or implant or hormonal coil) and is healthy, this cycle of oestrogen building then dropping at ovulation, followed by progesterone building then dropping to allow the bleed, continues throughout the fertile years of her life.

---

[1] *http://www.ncbi.nlm.nih.gov/pubmed/4053451*

Have all my eggs left the building, then?

It is a normal part of a woman's maturation that this cycling of oestrogen and progesterone will stop at some point in her life. The average age at which this occurs is 51-52 years. Exactly what triggers the change is not known. There is some evidence to suggest a genetic link, as women who are close blood relatives tend to begin the process at a similar age. There is also some evidence to suggest that initial menopausal symptoms start when the number of eggs a woman has left has fallen to 25,000. The reality is, it is not very well understood – slightly surprising, given that this is something that happens to 50% of the population!

Understanding that there are still eggs in the ovary, and that hormones are still active (if less reliable), makes it easier to realise that things don't come to an immediate stop. The hormone levels do not simply drop to nil. The ovaries do however produce less oestrogen as they becomes less functional.

Has all my oestrogen left the building, then?

There is more than one type of oestrogen. Why does this matter? During the reproductive years, the primary oestrogen hormone is a type called 17 beta-estradiol, which is produced in the ovaries. There are, though, other sources of oestrogen. The body still makes small amounts by a chemical process using an enzyme called aromatase. Aromatase is drawn from fatty tissue, and converts the androgens produced by the adrenal glands into oestrogen. These alternative sources are referred to as extragonadal (meaning outside of the sex organs).

So, no, all your oestrogen doesn't just leave the building as soon as menopausal symptoms hit. However, the other sources aren't as efficient as the ovaries, because the oestrogen has to go through a metabolic change to make it useable. This means that you might not get the full benefit.

As in puberty, fat is critical to synthesising appropriate levels of oestrogen, and therefore helps to keep the body in a healthy hormonal balance. This is why women tend to put on a little bit of weight around their waist at this time, as the body must have access to a healthy amount of fat in that area in order for the aromatase to form the oestrogen. This is not to say that being significantly overweight is healthy; but some larger ladies can make more oestrogen after their menopause than thinner ones who are still having fertile ovulatory cycles.

Many menopausal women experience weight gain and body-shape changes that seem suddenly out of control and out of proportion to their lifestyle – and we will come to that later in this book. We must all expect some changes as we age, but suffering such symptoms is certainly not a necessary part of the menopausal process.

As mentioned above, the menopause is a process of change that happens over time. In medical terminology, it is divided into two parts: peri-menopause and post-menopause.

Peri-menopause

The peri-menopause begins a few years before periods actually stop. One aspect of peri-menopause is a change in how well you mature and produce eggs – many women do not notice or frankly care about this, as the signs are quite subtle. The first indication you might get that you are entering this stage is increasing irregularity in the menstrual length. You might begin to notice a period being a couple of days late, perhaps, and the next a couple of days early; and gradually the timing becomes more erratic. The bleed might change a little too, becoming darker and drier.

The trigger for the start of the peri-menopause seems likely to be a gradual reduction in the number of ovarian follicles. A common misconception is that we 'run out' of eggs. For the sake of easy mathematics, let's assume that we menstruate for 40 years (say between age 10 and age 50), with 12 cycles per year. Given that one egg is released in each cycle, this accounts for only 480 eggs. Although the exact number of potential eggs (follicles) a woman is born with is unknown, it is estimated to be in the region of one to two million. At the time of puberty, it is estimated that a girl will have approximately 300,000 eggs.

Clearly the number of ovarian follicles that grow and mature into eggs decreases as we age. Some eggs are still in place, but we aren't able to mature them in the same way, and some naturally diminish and disappear. It seems more likely that it is a hormonal trigger that makes the follicles stop producing oestrogen and developing into eggs, rather than a lack of eggs that causes the hormones to drop away – although, as mentioned above, some studies indicate that a figure of about 25,000 eggs left seems significant for the start of peri-menopause, and 10,000 for menopause. (We'll avoid a chicken and egg joke here!) The evidence is not absolutely clear.

As peri-menopause progresses, the cycle can become even more erratic, as egg production becomes more erratic too.

Some women experience intermittent unusual flooding, or a bleed that isn't especially heavy but just continues for three to four weeks without stopping. This is due to the hormones that usually regulate the creation of the uterine lining, and serve as the 'start' and 'stop' signals for bleeding, not coming in in the usual way. In other words, the usual balanced cycle is changing.

The depletion of ovarian follicles (the natural reduction of eggs) leads to the variability of hormones normally produced by the ovary, which up till then will usually have been more predictable. This change in the way oestrogen is produced has repercussions throughout the body. It causes an increase in luteinising hormone (LH) and follicle stimulating hormone (FSH). A blood test can be run to look at the level of FSH. If this shows an increase, and the woman is aged 45-55 and possibly displaying a few symptoms, it is assumed that she is in peri-menopause.

Over the course of a year or so, these symptoms generally continue to progress, eventually leading to skipped periods and the cycle length becoming 60 days or more, until the bleed disappears altogether. During this stage, a woman might still be having ovulatory cycles (i.e. might still be producing eggs from the ovaries), but not reliably so. Fertility will drop very substantially, as many of the cycles will not be ovulatory; that is, they will not result in the ovary producing an egg, even though the hormones might have built a lining in the uterus and there might have been a bleed.

As peri-menopause progresses, the bleed becomes more erratic still, and the woman can experience some of the symptoms classically thought of as menopausal, such as hot flushes, sleep disturbance and mood-swings. Many women are told that they should expect this to last for anything from one to ten years. In truth, however, it should not be a long drawn-out process. The total time from the very first, almost imperceptible symptoms through to the final bleed should be no more than four years. There is no need for you to face unpleasant symptoms for an extended time, and you can take charge of your menopause.

In our clinic, once we rebalance a woman's hormones, we find that this part of her menopause hurries along nicely and ends quickly, or that normal ovulatory cycles resume for a couple of years until the body is completely ready to enter, go through and then exit this stage. We will come back to this later in the book, and give practical advice for helping the transition along.

Post-menopause

When you haven't had a bleed for a year, you have formally reached menopause. It is now considered safe for any contraception to be discontinued; if you have a coil, it can be removed. Unfortunately, though, the symptoms at this time can become worse, not better! We have met women whose symptoms have continued for over 15 years, and haven't really settled down.

\\

CASE STUDY – VICKI

'I'm an old bat and everyone hates me. I'm bad tempered, and have no patience with my family. I never seem

to settle or relax or sleep properly. I was fine before, but when I got hot flushes I became more irritable. I thought it would all settle down once the bleed stopped, but actually my moods and flushes just got worse. My husband has said, "You need to do something. I don't know what, but something!" So here I am – please help me feel normal again.'

Vicki had passed through menopause and her bleed had stopped for over a year, so her hormones should have settled. The fact that they hadn't indicated something wasn't right.

Her hormones hadn't settled correctly, so that had to be addressed. As it turned out, the homeopathic remedies Sepia and Chamomilla worked for Vicki; but herbal remedies such as sage and Bush Flowers could also have been effective. The most important thing to realise is that a state such as Vicki was in isn't a normal, acceptable one, and there are steps you can take to deal with it.

There are no clear official guidelines on how long the whole period of peri-menopause and post-menopause symptoms should last. The NHS suggests that the menopause should last from two to five years, but the latest advice from the government is that women can experience symptoms into their sixties or even their seventies. Symptoms continuing for such an extended period of time is a sign that things are out of kilter and need to be addressed, not passively accepted.

When women come to our clinic for help with the menopause, generally their symptoms are controlling them, and their lives are being shaped around the symptoms. Hot flushes are interrupting their work day and keeping them awake at night. Mood-swings, depression and lack of sleep are having a negative effect on their relationships and social lives. It is not at all uncommon for them to be experiencing anxiety, and they often report having panic attacks for the first time around this stage. Another almost universal complaint is an inability to control body weight and shape, despite diet and gym sessions.

We use homeopathy, along with some nutritional therapies, to treat clients in this situation, and this generally has immediate effects. Intrusive symptoms lessen considerably or disappear. Our conclusion, then, is that it isn't necessary simply to wait for the situation to resolve itself – and 10-15 years is an extraordinarily long chunk of your life for you to have to suffer through! It really shouldn't take that long.

Using the strategies and practical approaches described in the later chapters of this book, you can take charge of your life, and actually thrive through this important and exciting time.

Menopause is an exciting time – really?

Yes, the menopause is a time of creativity and new opportunities; a time of discovery. It is all about how you are, and what is important for you at this stage of your life. Although in this chapter we have started by looking at the physical aspect, it must be remembered that this is just one part of the process; the changes that take place are far more than just physical. We would be doing less than full justice to the subject of menopause if we were to limit and reduce it (and ourselves) to hormonal and physical symptoms.

Another really important aspect of this is the transition it represents, into a new phase of life. The menopause is the beginning of a new era, when the change in hormones releases us. No longer are we held in a monthly cycle of rising and falling oestrogen and progesterone levels; a cycle that switches our biology toward children and family over-responsibility, and that often causes us pain and makes us feel exhausted, angry, irritable and over-emotional – not to mention the inconvenience of the bleed itself. Now, instead, the brain biology is all about freedom; and women often say to us that this has become the most creative and happy time of their lives.

In many traditional societies, the older women are valued for their wisdom; they are the sages of their tribe. They have borne and raised children. They have experienced the problems and found solutions. They have coped with the difficulties of relationships and of managing a home and family. They have taken advantage of opportunities and made livelihoods, and seen both the potential benefits and the potential pitfalls.

This is the age of your wisdom; your age to fly.

The rest of this book will take a holistic view of the menopause, encompassing both the physical changes and the development that takes place on an emotional and spiritual level.

We will be presenting case studies showing how women, once they claim this experience, find themselves moving into a new space.

Summary

The menopause is a transition from one normal healthy state to another normal healthy state – it is not a loss.

The process starts with peri-menopause, when your body is prepared; progresses to menopause, when your monthly cycle finally stops; and ends with post-menopause, when you reach a new place of freedom.

The specifics of the menopause are not well understood. You can become the expert of your own menopause. The process should not take over years and years of your life; from the subtle, hardly noticeable beginnings to the end, it should last no more than four years.

As with all transitions, there is some degree of chaos; but you can learn the right way to manage the hormonal and emotional changes and flourish in your new place.

The menopause is a transition, not a 'stop'. It is not a pathology to be treated or suffered. We can remain well-balanced, strong and healthy if we make the process a smooth one, and the changes perfectly-timed.

2 MY PERIODS HAVE GONE A BIT CRAZY – WHAT IS HAPPENING?

Although changes to periods are often one of the first signs of menopause, they can be very subtle to start with, and nowhere near as dramatic as many women have been led to expect.

CASE STUDY – EMILY

'It was only when I started having hot flushes that I looked back over my periods for the last six months and realised that actually they had been coming either a few days early or a few days late, and that the bleed was a bit darker than before. I had expected that I would suddenly miss a month when the menopause came.'

This client had been experiencing symptoms that indicated she was in peri-menopause. As discussed in the previous chapter, this is a period of time when a woman's hormones begin to change. A drop in average progesterone levels and erratic oestrogen surges mean that egg maturation and ovulation become slightly less strong. Eventually the woman begins to get more noticeable physical symptoms, indicating that her body is definitely moving from fertility to post-fertility.

If you are someone who follows her cycle very carefully, and you know on which day you are due to begin your bleed, then you might notice a small difference at first, perhaps of only a day (either early or late). You might also notice a change in the quality or the length of bleed. Perhaps the blood is a little less fluid, or a little less red. Perhaps the heaviness is changing.

Shouldn't I just expect the bleed to decrease quite quickly and then stop?

This does happen in some cases, but it is a common misconception that the same is true for all women. Most experience it as a gradual process. Understanding your periods, and why any changes are taking place, can be very useful.

It is a big transition for the body to go through, moving from a time of fertility to a time of post-fertility. Prior to the menopause, it is doing all of the following things during each fertile cycle:

First two weeks

- boosting oestrogen;

- maturing an egg;

- ovulating;

- reducing and clearing oestrogen out of the system.

Second two weeks

- boosting progesterone;

- building uterine lining (endometrium);

- checking for fertilised egg;

- getting ready for possible pregnancy;

- clearing progesterone;

- bleed.

Then the cycle starts all over again.

The drop in the average level of progesterone at peri-menopause means that the uterine lining – which is what comes away during the bleed – changes quality. This is also influenced by fluctuations in oestrogen changing how well the egg is matured. The erratic levels of oestrogen in the body at this time mean that the cycles are no longer as smooth and predictable as in the past.

The following would be typical examples of early peri-menopausal cycles:

CYCLE ONE

- Lighter bleed for three days (before menopause this would have been five days);

- less mucus than normal throughout the month;

- bleed begins again after three weeks (before menopause this would have been four weeks).

CYCLE TWO

The next cycle has different characteristics:

- bleed for seven days;

- normal levels of mucus throughout the month;

- bleed begins again after five weeks.

The two cycles might continue alternating, or they might change, with the shorter one becoming shorter still (less than three weeks) and the longer one getting even longer (more than five weeks). The bleeding might also change and become shorter (less than three days) or longer (more than three days).

So, it is unpredictable?

'Unpredictable' is the key word here. You might have two or three lovely smooth cycles, followed by one erratic one where the hormones aren't as strong – or vice versa!

For some women, the change-over can be quick, for others, much slower and more gradual. However, it shouldn't go on for ages – most women can observe their cycles changing and then stopping over the course of about a year to 18 months. If this is not the case for you, it is worth first checking that all is well by visiting your doctor, and then looking at some of the alternative methods we describe later on to ensure that you pass smoothly through this phase, by boosting your body's natural ability to produce the correct hormonal signals to the brain and organs. You will feel better if your body is working better!

Sometimes, though, the unpredictability can go beyond just having erratic cycles.

CASE STUDY – LISA

'I had always been one of the lucky ones – my cycles had never really given me much trouble. But now suddenly I couldn't go anywhere anymore without worrying about having a period. Even when it wasn't fully there, it just never seemed to stop. My husband thought I was making it up to avoid him! When was this going to stop?'

As this case study illustrates, although the most common symptom women experience is erratic cycles, the bleed itself can become disrupted. It may be far heavier than usual, occasionally even flooding. In fact, far from stopping or becoming irregular, sometimes the bleed can just be very long or feel continuous. In extreme cases, it can be so extended and excessive as to cause anaemia. Other women have prolonged lighter bleeding or spotting – a frustrating and annoying occurrence. The nature of the blood flow can change too – becoming darker, or grainier and drier – although this might not be immediately obvious.

Why exactly do women experience symptoms like these?

Women are often told that when the peri-menopause begins they become oestrogen deficient, and that is why they experience such adverse symptoms. The truth, though, is that oestrogen levels are very variable, and can actually become extremely high during the peri-menopause. This is something that is generally overlooked in medical studies, as these tend to focus on the low measures found and ignore the high peaks – which can be even higher than those in young women at their most fertile.

To understand the full picture, it is necessary to consider the subtle interaction of several different hormones. Key factors in this are the level of follicle stimulating hormone (FSH); the level of inhibin hormone; and the balance between oestrogen and progesterone.

The function of FSH is to stimulate the ovaries to produce follicles and eggs. Inhibin, as the name suggests, is meant to stop an action; in this case, the action of the FSH. During the menopause, inhibin ceases to function in the way that it used to, so the FSH no longer has a cut-out. Therefore the FSH starts to increase and stimulates several follicles each cycle, rather than the usual single follicle. This makes the oestrogen levels higher and far more variable and volatile, while the progesterone levels are lower than before.

This unstable situation accounts for some of the most common symptoms that accompany peri-menopause: swollen, tender breasts (especially at the front); increased vaginal discharge; and a heavy, aching feeling in the abdomen. Likewise, heavy bleeding, frequent bleeding and extended spotting can all be a sign that oestrogen is too variable and progesterone too low. It is oestrogen that gives the signal for a woman's body to stop the bleed and prepare for a new egg and ovulation. The unpredictable nature of oestrogen production during the peri-menopause can mean that the signal either is not given, or is not received by the brain. Therefore endometrium goes on being produced and just comes away continually – a bit like trying to fill a wash-basin with the plug out! This is not a useful or necessary part of menopause.

For some women, the symptoms are of a relatively minor and/or transitory nature, but for others they can be debilitating and/or prolonged. There are natural differences between individuals – some people are quicker at getting over colds or recovering from a trip, for instance, and some children grow quicker or slower than others, or in spurts. However, the key thing to bear in mind is that your body should be progressing in this process – too often it gets stuck and the symptoms become problematic.

Knowing yourself is a good start. Ask yourself:

• Does my body tends to adapt more quickly or more slowly?

• How strong and settled have my hormones been throughout my life?

• How quickly did my periods establish themselves when they first started?

These are useful indicators to yourself as to whether or not the process is progressing as quickly as it should be. It is worth repeating, though, that symptoms should not be so bad as to affect the quality of your life. If they are, this might indicate that your hormones are not shifting properly and are going out of balance. The body's natural state is to be in balance, and it will always try to create that. A passing phase when it seems to be out of balance – perhaps one bad period followed by a much better one – can simply indicate that the body is learning to change; it is progressing and travelling through the journey of menopause. But a continued difficult state suggests that it might need a bit of help.

So, what can a woman in this situation do?

Where erratic cycles are concerned, there are homeopathic remedies that can address the issue, as well as other natural approaches that can be helpful. This is something we discuss in more detail a little later on. If the problem is simply one of oestrogen levels, it should respond reasonably quickly, often within one or two cycles.

If there is excessive or unusual bleeding, it can be worth first of all getting some simple tests done to rule out anything medically wrong. Hormone tests, ultrasound scans or even an examination of the uterus (a hysteroscopy) or an endometrial biopsy might be suggested.

A hormone test is a simple blood test, and is a useful way of assessing if you are peri-menopausal or even in full menopause. A full blood test can also pick up some other issues e.g. thyroid problems. Always ask your doctor for the actual results; being assured that everything is 'fine' or 'normal' actually tells you very little! Are the results normal for menopause? Are they normal for peri-menopause? Much as some healthcare professionals worry that clients will misinterpret results, women have the right to be fully informed of their own health and take charge of their lives!

An ultrasound scan involves placing a small probe inside the vagina and angling it so that the cervix, uterus, ovaries and any growths in the fallopian tubes can be visualised.

A hysteroscopy essentially involves having a look inside the uterus/womb with a camera. It also allows for a sample of the uterus to be taken (endometrial biopsy). This is invasive but does give more information than an ultrasound scan.

Often an ultrasound scan or a hysteroscopy will show nothing of great concern. Sometimes, though, women can be given news that seems worrying; fibroids, polyps, endometrial thickening (thickening of the lining of the womb) or cysts might be seen. In such cases, it is easy to presume that whatever has been seen is the cause of any symptoms, and that its removal would help. That might not be the case, however. The findings could be incidental – that is, unrelated to any symptoms you are experiencing – and you could end up going through surgery for little benefit.

The detection of fibroids usually reflects normal peri-menopausal changes rather than pathological changes. Fibroids are a symptom of hormonal imbalances that have got out of control; they are produced by excess hormones drifting around the body. This can happen at any time in a woman's life when either hormone levels are erratic or the body is producing an excess of one hormone over another. However, the menopause is a time when this is particularly likely to occur, because of the natural hormonal fluctuations involved. These fluctuations can cause the fibroids to grow.

Fibroids are often difficult to remove, and removing them doesn't get to the root cause of the problem – i.e. the erratic hormones – so they often come back again. Their growth can be controlled by rebalancing the hormones. This causes them to shrink and not regrow – it is as if their 'food supply' has been taken away!

If you do get medical tests done, remember to ask lots of questions when you receive the results. Don't assume that surgery is the only option to tackle any issues that might be identified. Consider if simply waiting and seeing is appropriate, or if other steps to tackle your hormone imbalance could work. Think whether or not the results actually make sense.

Won't the pill or the coil stave off nasty menopausal bleed symptoms?

There is a misconception that if you stay on a hormonal method of contraception until you are way over the usual menopausal age, and then discontinue it, the menopause will just be there – no peri-menopausal symptoms, no unpleasant hot flushes. You just bypass the whole thing, surely? Sadly not. If this were the case, we would certainly be recommending it!

In fact, the body has to adapt and change – there is no shortcut. It has to move from one state – fertile with menstrual cycle – to another – infertile with no cycle. As previously explained, this involves changing how it produces hormones – especially oestrogen, which shifts from being produced in high amounts from the ovaries to lesser amounts from adrenal and fat cells. A natural, gradual process is needed for this.

If you are taking synthetic hormones such as the contraceptive pill, or having hormone replacement therapy (HRT), suddenly stopping these can cause a sharp change in the body. This can actually exacerbate undesirable symptoms, as the menopause comes in with a bang – there has been no gradual handover.

We have also seen clients who have menopausal symptoms despite still being on the pill or having a hormonal coil. The synthetic hormones that are put into the body by these contraceptive methods can keep the body in a stable routine. However, once menopause begins, the body's natural hormones become erratic. The stable synthetic hormones are now pushing against the erratic natural hormones, the levels of which can be either high or low at different times. This can cause worse mood-swings, spots, bleeding or a general feeling of being a bit unwell.

If you are used to using a hormonal method of contraception, it is very useful to consider well in advance what approach might suit you when you reach menopausal age – otherwise you might find a surprise you didn't really reckon on!

I've always had bad periods, so I'm looking forward to the menopause

The idea that the menopause can bring relief from bad periods is another common misconception. If you generally suffer heavy or painful periods, or severe mood-swings, it is very likely that you have somewhat out-of-balance hormones; and unfortunately that can mean that you will have a more difficult menopause. When women come to see us with heavy and/or painful periods or mood-swings, we give treatments aimed at balancing their hormones, and we generally see their symptoms disappear.

Menopause is a time of change and erratic hormones, so if this comes on top of an already unbalanced menstrual cycle, more often than not it causes symptoms to become worse and not better. So it's good idea to take steps in advance to make sure that your menstrual cycle is as good as it can be. If you consult your doctor about this, you might find you are offered progesterone hormone therapy, or a hormonal coil, or a hysteroscopy. Progesterone hormone therapy is a type of HRT taken during the second half of the cycle. For some women this can offer some relief and reduce bleed; but if your hormones are not naturally balanced, it does nothing to address that, and you might need to consider alternative measures in the future. The hormonal coil is often suggested to help with heavy bleeding as it incorporates progesterone. In our experience this rarely proves helpful and often leads to increased painful bleeding and greater mood changes and instability. As described above, hysteroscopy essentially involves having a look inside the uterus/womb with a camera, and also allows for an endometrial biopsy to be taken. As with any medical tests, make sure that you are fully informed of any options presented to you when you get the results. Remember that while it is possible to remove any fibroids etc by surgery, this doesn't necessarily mean that it is the best option for you personally.

Can I do anything myself to help get through this?

Many symptoms will settle naturally as the peri-menopause continues – progression and improvement are the key things to look for. You shouldn't be stuck at this stage of changes. If symptoms aren't too troublesome, and you develop an action plan following the advice in this book on diet, exercise and so on, this could be sufficient.

If you feel that more is required, our recommendation would be that you explore natural therapies, then wait and see, and reassess how these are working for you. Most symptoms will have come to the fore because of erratic hormones, so it is certainly worth trying to rebalance your hormones naturally.

If symptoms do not respond to self-help, you might consider seeing a professional who is qualified in a natural therapy that you would like to try. They will have access to more powerful aspects of that therapy.

Always have persistently troublesome symptoms checked by a doctor.

What natural therapies could I try?

Possible approaches to try are:

- Topical hormonal therapy. Progesterone cream is available over-the-counter, and a small, pea-sized amount can be rubbed into fatty areas (e.g. thigh or stomach). Many women find this helpful to balance hormones. Wild Yam cream can also be used.

- Homeopathic treatment. While many remedies are possible, it is worth trying one of the most common in the first instance. Take Sepia and Folliculinum 200c twice daily at the start of a bleed, and if this is the appropriate remedy, it should reduce and shorten the bleed within two cycles. Carcinosin and Calcium Carbonate are sometimes good additional supports; Carcinosin is particularly useful for women with a tendency to overextend themselves, while Calcium Carbonate is indicated for women who have very heavy bleeding and do not take easily to the thought of change. Do see a professional homeopath if this doesn't help, as a different remedy might be required.

- Herbal support. Herbal remedies can be enormously helpful. The most common one used for irregular and heavy peri-menopausal bleeding is Agnus Castus. Source a good-quality version. There are many other herbal options, and if this hasn't helped sufficiently, it might be worth seeing a qualified medical herbalist, who will be able to provide individualised herbal treatment.

- Alfalfa. This is a good supplement to take for problems with bleeding.

- Vitamins. Multi-vitamin tablets with high levels of Vitamins B, C, E and D are useful. Always ensure that any vitamins you take are high-quality and food-state – that is, manufactured from foods rather than chemicals.

CASE STUDY – JANET

'My periods were never light, but my God they went crazy once I turned 48! I was flooding so much that I couldn't actually leave the house for two days. This couldn't go on – I was just exhausted and miserable. The doctor had

suggested endometrial ablation, and if that didn't work a hysterectomy, all of which seemed a bit scary and drastic.

Anne and Claire saw me, and I said I would give them three months to treat this, or I would have to bite the bullet and have surgery, just so I could get on with my life. They did a pretty good job, using homeopathic treatments and herbal supplements. The periods did get to be more manageable, and I felt so much better. No surgery, and now I am almost through to the other side, hopefully to be period-free very shortly!'

Summary

Heavy and unusual bleeds are actually a normal symptom during menopause but can be extremely disruptive and troublesome. They are a result of hormonal disturbances, and should be easily and quickly helped with natural treatment. You do not have to put up with them.

Symptoms should be transient, and progress quickly toward normalising.

If you are concerned, get your doctor to check that there is nothing unusual happening. The tests that can be undertaken are fairly straightforward procedures, but can be invasive. Once you have the results, you have a choice about dealing with the symptoms. You do not have to continue just to 'suffer' with them, or to take medication if you want to try something different – you have options.

If your cycles have been difficult during your fertile

years, it is likely that the menopause will cause more unwelcome symptoms rather than fewer. It is worth taking steps to balance your hormones and life before the menopause hits.

3 HAS MENOPAUSE REALLY BEGUN? AND WHAT DOES IT MEAN FOR MY FERTILITY?

Once the menopause starts, can I delay it and get back to my normal periods?

The short answer is no. But often we see that women who are stressed, and busy juggling many different responsibilities at this time of their life, find their menopause starting a bit early. Perhaps they have teenage children, or elderly parents, who can be demanding. Perhaps they are getting used to life or job changes. Or perhaps they are just worn out from chasing their tails for twenty years!

CASE STUDY – MARY

'I came to see Anne and Claire to sort out my hot flushes. My bleed was odd, so I thought I was menopausal. I'm 47, so it wasn't entirely unexpected. I wanted to just make sure I got through things as naturally as possible, especially as I have a youngish child and a busy life. I was quite surprised when the homeopathic remedies brought back my normal cycle and got rid of all the hot flushes. Seems like I've a couple of years to go yet.'

In cases such as this, it seems that the hormones, which are becoming more variable and a touch chaotic, have problems re-adjusting, and therefore produce peri-menopausal symptoms a bit earlier than is really necessary. In our clinic, we see many women who are aged about 45-50, have irregular cycles and simply assume they are menopausal. Sometimes they have had a blood test indicating that they are in or approaching the early stages of peri-menopause. However, this might not be the whole story. The body might be prematurely changing toward a menopausal state.

Certainly where we have treated clients such as Mary (case study above) with simple homeopathic remedies such as Sepia and Folliculinum, and perhaps a constitutional remedy, we have seen clear changes to their cycle; it has become more regular again. Subsequent blood tests have shown that the level of follicle stimulating hormone (FSH) has dropped, meaning that the woman is not quite ready yet to enter peri-menopause. This might still be one to three years away.

Holistic therapy improves the body's response to stress and illness, helps the hormones work better, and can put the menopause back to its correct time – but not unnaturally beyond it!

Am I genuinely menopausal, or could it be something else?

CASE STUDY – LINDA

'I've had a terrible two years, what with one thing and

another. I really wanted another baby, and I usually fall pregnant quickly, but that hasn't happened this time. My periods are all over the place. I'm only 32, but my doctor has just told me that my FSH level is the same as a menopausal woman's. I had my last baby only two years ago. Can this change happen so quickly?'

In this case, the test results seemed not to make sense. Linda had no symptoms, was very young and had recently had a baby. The results were more indicative of a woman in her fifties who had been experiencing noticeable menopausal symptoms and whose last baby had been born much longer ago. What was happening?

When Linda came to see us, she told us that she had had a lot of changes and challenges in her life since having her last child. Her blood test had indeed shown a very high FSH level, which in most circumstances would have been indicative of peri-menopause. However, after we had treated her for two months with homeopathy and natural supplements, Linda had another test done that showed her FSH level was back to normal. This held for a while until she had another difficult life event, followed by further stress. Then her FSH level was once again found to be high. It was clear to us that Linda's hormone levels were severely affected by stress. Once she turned her attention to relieving that stress, her FSH level normalised fully.

In Linda's case, it didn't really make sense to consider her initial test result as being indicative of a natural early menopause. It is always worth bearing in mind the complete picture, and having a repeat test if you think you might be in a similar situation.

At least, now my periods are changing, I don't have to worry about getting pregnant!

Not true! While at this stage in their lives most women are no longer ovulating as regularly as they once did, ovulation (and therefore potentially conception) can still occur until menopause is clearly established – which is considered to be one full year after the last bleed.

There is a common misconception that after the age of 40 a woman is very unlikely to conceive; an often quoted statistic puts the chance at 20%. This is based on very old data, and doesn't actually represent what is going on in today's world. Abortion rates of women over 40 currently exceed those of younger girls.

Women in their late forties often consider themselves 'safe' from pregnancy, and don't bother to renew their pill prescription or have their coil or implant replaced when it reaches the end of its life, thinking that contraception is no longer really needed. This is a false assumption.

We had one client, who hadn't had a bleed for the past three months, suddenly find that she had ovulated and happened to conceive. A real surprise for both her and her partner – although actually, once they got used to the idea, they and their grown-up children were happy!

In our fertility clinic we see a lot of women aged over 40 who are wanting to have a baby, and usually it isn't their age in itself that we have found to be blocking the conception.

More commonly it is out-of-balance hormones, stress, anxiety, exhaustion or what we tend to call 'wear, tear and depreciation'. In other words, it can be just because they have so much going on in their work and home lives, or because they have had a cold or other illness that has left them feeling less than 100%. Money concerns; DIY; even organising a holiday can create stress! Being older means we have more to carry in our life, and stress can affect all of our body systems, including our hormones.

Some women are particularly sensitive to the effects of the types of synthetic hormones that come in the contraceptive pill, implant or hormonal coil, or to the drugs used in IVF treatment. Consequently, unlike many other women who are able simply to bounce back, they can feel that their health and energy have never been quite the same since having these medications. Different people's bodies cope with drug treatments in different ways; some take a long time to overcome their effects, others less so.

There are many factors that affect fertility, apart from age, so if you are at a stage in your life where you are happily looking forward to not having children, it is a good idea for you to continue to use contraception until a complete year has passed since your last period. Natural contraception, such as a barrier method or the copper coil, is preferable too. Using a hormonal method such as the pill, a coil, an implant or an injection will get in the way of the natural rebalancing that is necessary to pass through menopause. Keep a note of your bleeds. Then you will be able to keep track of how you are progressing and how things are changing; and most importantly you will know when a year has passed since the last bleed and it is 'safe' to stop contraception.

Summary

Menopausal symptoms can sometimes start a little earlier than is really necessary; but menopause cannot be turned back by natural methods once it has genuinely begun.

Homeopathic remedies can be good way of ensuring that the body begins the process at the right time.

Make sure you continue with contraception until at least one year after your last bleed, as you can still be fertile!

4 HOT FLUSHES

Of all the symptoms of menopause, hot flushes or hot flashes are the most common, and for many women the most dreaded.

Case Study – Karen

'My life now revolves around having a stack of towels by the side of the bed. I sleep on one, and an hour or so later wake up, soaking wet and desperate to cool down any way I can. The towel is soaking wet too. I dry myself and put a new towel under me. I do this all night. I can't go on like this. I'm not sleeping, I'm fed up, it's not sexy and my washing machine is going to give up on me soon! Is this really normal?'

Not everyone has such extreme and debilitating symptoms as Karen, but unfortunately many women do have serious, uncomfortable and at times embarrassing hot flushes. We have had clients who suffer almost as badly as Karen during the day, and this can affect job performance and career, as well as being extremely unpleasant. As one client described it, 'How can I do a big presentation when I'm dripping all over and red in the face? It can catch you unawares and almost always at the worst moment. I feel quite powerless.'

Because you are unable to predict the timing of hot flushes, or the severity of them, or do anything about them when they arrive, they can make you feel completely out of control. Being so physically uncomfortable can also make you feel very self-conscious.

In this chapter we will discuss the symptoms of hot flushes in some depth, and look at why they might be happening. But the crucial thing to realise is: you do not need to suffer from them.

Some women have only the occasional hot flush – perhaps one or two during the day and a couple at night – and this is a normal part of them passing through menopause. But being out of control, and having life-limiting symptoms, is not. It is important to find the right solutions to combat this, not just because you want to enjoy life to the full, but also because having balanced hormones enables the menopause to pass quickly into a joyous post-menopausal phase.

What do hot flushes feel like?

Hot flushes are experienced differently from person to person, but have some common characteristics, especially when they are problematic.

The hot feeling itself is usually very different from that of being in a hot environment, such as a room with a blazing fire, or a tropical climate. The heat is intense and sudden, and you can feel as if your skin is on fire, or you are burning deep on the inside. It begins internally, and is usually very quick and uncontrolled. There can be a sensation of flashing, or of burning, sometimes accompanied by profuse sweating, and a feeling of being completely unable to cool down without taking action. It can be overwhelming and distressing. Some women, after being so hot, can then suddenly feel absolutely freezing. It is as if their body temperature gauge doesn't work properly anymore, and is going crazy!

Hot flushes at night can be particularly problematic. They can be more extreme than during the day; and of course they inevitably disturb your sleep! In addition, they can result in you being sweaty, even running with sweat, quite unlike during the day – as in Karen's case, some women have to change their bedding or nightwear regularly. Night-time flushes also seem to be more persistent than daytime ones, and once woken by them, many women find it difficult to get back to sleep again.

Hot flushes don't always pass quickly; they can stick around, and lead to a feeling of getting hotter and hotter, unless some kind of remedial action is taken. A lot of women choose to use a fan, but others find this insufficient and have to take more extreme measures such as applying cold flannels or towels, or standing outside in cold weather, in order to feel cooler again. This often results in a pendulum action, with the feeling of being too hot followed by one of being too cold; and it can also impact on the husband or partner, who sometimes starts to think that they will never again have a warm night with the window closed!

In fact, this inability to control temperature is probably the most prevalent, and also one of the earliest, signs of the hormone changes that run throughout peri-menopause and beyond.

For some women, these flushes are not just physically disruptive. They can be accompanied by a strange sensation of feeling 'odd', or of being anxious when you haven't been before; just not yourself.

With some women experiencing these symptoms many times, both during the day and at night, this is disruptive and can affect their ability to live a normal life.

Understanding your hot flushes

The exact cause of hot flushes is not known. However, this is what we do know.

All our menstrual hormones are controlled through the action of the part of the brain called the hypothalamus. This is the control centre for the hormones, and for how they affect other parts of the body. The hypothalamus is also responsible for regulating and maintaining a constant bodily temperature. It is likely that part of the cause of hot flushes is a disruption in the flow of chemical messages to and from the hypothalamus, affecting its ability to maintain a stable temperature. However, this is not the whole story. There is a complex system at work.

In the earlier chapters we described how during peri-menopause the body is beginning to access some oestrogen in a different way; not solely using the ovaries, but instead metabolising by way of the adrenal system and fat tissues. The oestrogen harvested here is harder for the body to release and has to go through a chemical process before it can be used. All metabolic processes such as this release heat, so this might also be part of the picture.

Why are hot flushes so unpredictable?

There is a common misconception that menopause consists of nothing more than a reduction in oestrogen levels. In fact, as noted previously, high levels of oestrogen have been observed in women who are in the early stages of menopause. Rather than actually going low or staying high, the levels are variable and unstable - and they remain so until menopause is fully complete.

The body is trying to balance and manage these constantly shifting, far less stable hormones. It seems it is often unable to keep up with the swings and changes – leading to a sudden excess or lack of certain hormones and consequent temperature shifts.

An example of how unstable things can be at this time is that a woman can still have an ovulatory cycle (i.e. produce an egg from the ovary) with an apparently normal bleed after not having done so for perhaps a few months previously. Then, she might not have another cycle again. That is a very changeable picture; no wonder the hormones are confused!

A rollercoaster of hormones

Women experience a 'rollercoaster' in oestrogen production at this time.

Before the start of any menopausal symptoms, women during their cycle regularly produce both oestrogen and follicular stimulating hormone (FSH). These stimulate the ovary to produce and mature an egg. When the egg is produced (ovulation) the body then releases an inhibitor hormone to tell it to stop producing FSH because the job is done – the egg is ready. Once peri-menopause begins, however, a couple of things happen that upset this settled picture. First, the level of the inhibitor hormone reduces. This means that the natural rise in FSH that is trying to stimulate the ovulation of an egg will have nothing to stop it continuing. Consequently the level of FSH becomes high. Once the FSH rises out of control in this way, it can cause an over-stimulation of the ovary, leading to unstable levels of oestrogen. Instead of oestrogen rising for the first half of the cycle, peaking and then dropping, there is a tendency for it too to keep pushing upward.

Adding to the instability is the fact that the ovaries are not maturing eggs in the way they used to. This means that sometimes they are under-producing oestrogen, and at other times over-producing.

The body is attempting to control and balance, and it does – but as on a rollercoaster, there are times in between when everything feels very out of control. Balance is particularly difficult to achieve because of the way the body is creating oestrogen from other sources. It is no wonder we have some swinging moods and symptoms!

It's not just oestrogen that's a problem

Alongside the muddle of the unstable oestrogen and FSH, we also have the progesterone situation! The progesterone level normally rises after ovulation, in the second half of the cycle. It reaches a peak and then drops just before the bleed, causing the bleed to start. During the peri-menopause, however, progesterone is not as regularly produced and maintained as it once was, and consequently the bleeding becomes erratic. In addition, the fall in the average level of progesterone has a knock-on effect on other hormones, particularly oestrogen.

Progesterone normally does the job of helping to balance the impact of oestrogen. If there is an excess of oestrogen in the body, progesterone helps to stabilise this. The way it does this is by making the sites where oestrogen is taken up (oestrogen receptors) less available, blocking it from being absorbed by the body, so that the excess is just excreted as a waste product.

In other words, when the progesterone level is in balance, it helps the body by keeping the level of oestrogen correct. If the progesterone becomes out of balance, as happens during peri-menopause, it can't do this job as effectively anymore. This in turn can cause:

- increased anxiety;

- sleeplessness;

- weight gain, especially around the waist; and

- loss of sex drive.

Other possible negative effects are less obvious but potentially more serious. These include increased insulin levels, and decreased insulin sensitivity (i.e. decreased ability to use insulin), with attendant risks of diabetes.

Variable progesterone levels are part of the hormonal rollercoaster observed in peri-menopausal women. However, once the post-menopausal phase is reached, progesterone levels remain stable and low.

Men have hot flushes too!

Many people are surprised to learn that men can also have hot flushes and sweats. This is most often observed in men who are having drug therapy or surgery that affects their testosterone levels, e.g. prostate cancer treatment.

This again demonstrates how hot flushes are related to the body losing key sex hormones (whether oestrogen or testosterone), and this in turn causing fluctuations and imbalance.

Do I have to suffer these symptoms?

Some outward sign that hormonal changes are happening is a natural thing. It would be strange if such important and profound changes were to occur without any indication at all. However, the symptoms do not need to be disruptive or life-changing.

One way of looking at the situation is to liken it to the beginning of your fertile years, when your periods first stated. Just as that change was probably a profound one for you, and made you feel quite different – having to get used to a new routine, with a physical bleed, mood changes and a sense of growing into womanhood – so the menopause marks the advent of the next stage of your hormonal life. This time, it is all about growing into your maturity and wisdom, into your freedom.

Symptoms such as hot flushes might be evident for a time, but should not be extreme, and should soon reduce until they are minimal. Becoming ensnared in them means that the process is stuck and not passing as it should.

We have noted above that hot flushes at night might stick around a little bit longer than daytime ones. Nobody knows precisely why this is, but from a holistic perspective, night-time is when the liver cleanses and detoxifies the body's metabolic processes, including the hormones. So, having a few hot flushes at night, provided that they wake you only briefly, are not especially sweaty, and can be quickly relieved by, say, sticking your foot out of bed to cool down, is actually a good sign that a change is taking place relatively well. Some women have found using a cooling blanket at night useful – these are specially designed blankets that are cool when first put on the body, and cool back down again naturally when you take them off, so can be used throughout the night if you need to from time to time.

Recently there have been reports that some women have hot flushes that go on into their sixties, their seventies or even their eighties! This need not happen. Symptoms persisting for that long simply means that the hormonal changes haven't resolved and settled as they should naturally do.

So, waiting for the hot flushes of menopause to pass, in the same way as one might wait for a cold to clear, is not always the right approach. These symptoms shouldn't be prolonged, and if they threaten to become so, you should look to see what action you can take to change the situation.

So, what can be done?

The first thing to remember is that the menopause is a change and a process – you cannot move through to the other side without experiencing some symptoms. However, you do not have to suffer! You do not have to grin and bear it! There are many things that will help the hormones to balance quickly, and as with menarche (your first period), you should pass through this stage as seamlessly as possible.

Relax!

Yes, really. Relaxing does help with hot flushes. Breathing slowly and calmly, and not allowing any panic or angry feelings to overtake you, is really important. If a hot flush strikes out of the blue, it can be a quite natural response to want to rush into action to try to 'fix' the feelings – by opening a window perhaps, or fanning yourself wildly in a panic. However, these apparent solutions can actually be counterproductive. The feeling of panic stimulates the adrenals and gets everything moving quickly, switching on the body's 'fight or flight mechanism' and thereby stimulating adrenaline and other hormones, pumping the blood hard and making the whole situation worse.

Meditation and mindfulness

Learning to meditate, doing yoga and deep breathing can all be extremely useful ways of helping to allow the hot flush sensations just to pass over you.

Homeopathic remedies

There is good evidence that homeopathy can be effective in treating hot flushes. A French randomised control, double blind trial (the same standard as used for pharmaceutical drugs) tested the efficacy of a commonly-used, non-hormonal homeopathic combination remedy for hot flushes against a placebo. It found that the remedy had significant and clear effects far in excess of the placebo.

There are many possible homeopathic remedies for hot flushes, but before approaching a professional homeopath there are some common ones that you can buy and are worth trying for yourself:

- Sepia 200 – A good general hormone balancer – particularly if there is low mood, low sex drive and lack of motivation. A good all-rounder.

- Carcinosin 200 – The second most common remedy for hot flushes, often indicated for women with a strong emotional picture of over-caring and over-responsibility.

- Folliculinum 200 – Another good general hormone balancer; it combines well with Sepia.

- Glonoinum 200 – Good for very hot flushes that are very sudden and can be accompanied by severe headaches, or flushes more in the face and head.

- Amyl Nit 200 – Good for very hot, extreme burning sensation that often comes from the centre of the chest upwards to the head.

- Sulph 20**0** – Good for use if sweaty, particularly if worse at night and your sleep is disrupted, or if the hair or hairline is sweaty or extremely hot.

Homeopathic remedies should be taken on a neutral palate and dissolved in the mouth. They can be taken as needed; one tablet up to six times a day if helpful. If no relief is felt after three days, then it is likely you will need one of the many other available remedies from a professional homeopath.

Herbal remedies

There are a wide range of herbal remedies available over-the-counter and on the internet. These have been used for many years for symptomatic relief, and you can consider trying them for perhaps a month to determine whether or not they are of help to you. Some herbs can have interactions with other medications, so do check with your pharmacist or doctor before taking them.

- Sage has long been used to deal with hot flushes that have a great deal of sweat involved. It is a good general menopause balancing herb.

- Black Cohosh is considered more indicated when there are mood-swings as well as hot flush symptoms.

Herbal remedies can be used alongside homeopathic ones if you would like to mix and match. If those mentioned above do not work for you, again there are many others available, but you should contact a professional herbalist for treatment.

Supplements, vitamins etc

This can be one of the most confusing and frustrating areas for women. If you walk into your local health food shop, you could easily feel overwhelmed by the choices available, and confused by the promises made on the packaging of the various products on sale. We recommend always taking food-state vitamins – those that have been manufactured from foods rather than chemicals – as these are fully absorbed and utilised by the body.

- Multi-vitamin is appropriate for women over 50. This should be food-state, with high levels of Vitamins B, C, D and E, plus chromium and magnesium.

- Magnesium on its own is another good choice. Ideally this should be food-state, and in a mix with calcium and Vitamin D for good bone support during this time.

- Fish oil, Krill oil, Evening Primrose oil and Flaxseed oil are all good for hormonal support. It is important to take good, high quality oils – especially in the case of fish oils, as poor quality fish oils can contain pollutants, including mercury.

- Magnesium oil is a good topical application; that is, a treatment applied externally to the skin.

A combination of these key things is in our experience sufficient for most women during menopause. Again, they can be combined with other approaches.

Diet

Your diet is important for your general health, and never more so than at the time of the menopause, when your body is going through amazing changes. But this does not mean that it is necessary for everyone to attempt extreme dietary changes. Overall, alkali-producing foods are important, because they reduce the risk of osteoporosis. Key points to remember are:

- Eating 60-120g of pulses and beans three times a week can elevate the phyto-oestrogens, which can help to reduce hot flushes and sweats.

- Increasing your intake of fruit, vegetables and grains (such as quinoa) can be helpful.

- Some people find that reducing coffee and alcohol intake helps, as these can be stimulating and therefore stimulate hot flushes.

- Papaya and flaxseeds can be very useful.

Summary

Hormones become very disordered and unstable during menopause. It is normal to have some transitory symptoms, but these shouldn't be so severe or prolonged as to be really troublesome.

Mild night flushes are not a cause for concern, provided that they are not disturbing your sleep too much. They are normal and should pass and improve within a year.

You do not need to grin and bear hot flushes that affect your life quality. There are many things you can do to help yourself.

Be proactive in taking steps to balance your hormones. This will help your body to readjust as quickly as possible and pass through this stage.

Homeopathy, herbs, vitamins and diet can all have a place in helping to minimise hot flushes.

5 ANXIETY, MOOD-SWINGS AND BAD SLEEP

CASE STUDY - ANDREA

'I'm feeling anxious and jittery. On top of that, I'm not sleeping. Is this coincidence, worry about getting older, or actually the menopause (or all of these!) Surely menopause is just a physical change?'

Menopause is physical, that's true. However, it is also chemical, hormonal and emotional. These are all interrelated. People are not just isolated physical beings. A change at one level can have a knock-on impact on every other. This is especially true during menopause, where the physical and chemical changes are radical.

In this part of the book we explore the really important emotional changes that so many women experience and haven't been able to explain. Women are often told that this is just part of ageing, or a separate issue – perhaps depression – especially if this is coinciding with other life events such as children leaving home, work pressures or other stresses. Little credence is given to the idea that the emotional changes they are experiencing are due to them being menopausal.

The good news is that there is a lot that women can do to alleviate anxiety, mood-swings or stressful feelings by natural means, without having to resort to medication or simply being told to 'suck it up'. If the cause is menopausal, there is so much that women can do to take charge of their life, feel in control again and not overwhelmed.

Women are often warned that the menopause will cause them to 'suffer' physical symptoms (hot flushes, erratic bleeds and weight gain), but are generally not told that other symptoms can include mood-swings and feelings of anxiety and panic. Consequently, particularly if they have few (or no) physical symptoms, they can often fail to realise that these emotional symptoms are in fact part of menopause, and not a sign that they are unable to cope.

The women we see in our clinic sometimes confess to being almost embarrassed, because they feel they ought to be coping better. They are surprised when they learn this is part of their menopause, and feel loads better once they begin addressing the imbalances that accompany the change they are going through.

Emotional mood-swings or feelings of panic and anxiety might arise on their own at this time, or might come in tandem with physical symptoms. It can really make women feel very unwell when they have both together. It is important to remember here that it is not necessary to suffer. It is possible to find things to help; and taking charge to find what works for you is an important part of this transition.

Anxiety

Not everyone does suffer anxiety at this time – it is not a required part of menopause! However, it can strike unexpectedly, and can range from the subtle – perhaps a slight lack of assurance – to the sudden, complete and life-changing.

A good example, which is quite typical, is a loss of confidence in the ability to drive. Strong, capable women who have previously driven all over the country and even travelled overseas without a thought can experience a weird, unexpected change.

CASE STUDY – SANDRA

'I hate getting into my car now. I just hate driving. I get so anxious if I have to turn right! Unbelievably for me, I can't contemplate going on a motorway. What the heck is going on! I used to be a medical sales rep, for goodness sake. There isn't a motorway I haven't been up and down without so much as a thought! What has happened to me?'

Anxiety as a menopausal symptom is often overlooked. All too often it is treated as a sign of stress or depression. Yes, it is true that women at this age are often having to cope with family or other stresses, such as teenage children, elderly parents or busy work life. But we have often found that there is a hormonal base to the anxiety, which actually arises from the menopause.

Getting on top of the hormonal changes can often cause the anxiety to dissipate – which is very freeing, allowing the woman to resume living her life normally (like Sandra being able to turn right at a junction again!) Everything is better when your hormones are in balance!

If the hormone imbalance is missed or ignored, some women can find they are given antidepressants or antianxiety medication, which not only fails to address the underlying cause, but can also reinforce the sense of feeling out of control, unable to cope and possibly unwell. The problems with medication are:

• you are reliant on the medication (if it works);

• you haven't changed or even addressed the underlying cause of your symptoms;

• you need a plan on how you are going to come off the medication safely;

• all medication has side-effects.

Women can be written off, and made to feel a bit silly and less capable as a person than they used to be. All their collected wisdom and experience is suddenly reduced to, 'Well, you are getting older, so perhaps you should slow down a bit,' with a pill prescribed to quieten the symptoms. None of which is asking, 'Is there an underlying cause?'

Sandra didn't realise that the menopause could make her feel this way – unfortunately, nor do many other women.

She was really relieved to discover that she wasn't losing her marbles. Once she understood that this was a passing phase rather than a permanent problem, she completely took charge of things and did everything possible, using a combination of homeopathic remedies, dietary changes to reduce processed foods and carbohydrates, and mindfulness meditation. This enabled the natural menopausal process to proceed as well and as quickly as possible – it was completed in about a year. Recognising that the root cause was her hormones, and that she wasn't going mad, made her feel in control again.

So, what are the choices and solutions for women who feel that they are unable to deal with situations that they used to cope with well? What if they are feeling generally anxious for no good reason? The following can all be of help:

- **Bach Flower remedies.** Rescue Remedy; Larch for loss of confidence; Aspen for feeling anxious and not knowing why.

- **Bush Flower remedies.** Calm and Clear is a special combination readily available online.

- **Homeopathic remedies.** A good anxiety treatment sold by the homeopathic pharmacies is Triple A, a combination of three remedies specially prepared to help with that 'panic'-type feeling. Additionally, health food shops will often stock Arsenicum Album, which is a good treatment for anxiety; Gelsemium, which is a good treatment for worry about what might possibly happen; Calc Carb, which can help with worry about change; and Nux Vomica, which is also good for anxiety.

- **Herbal remedies.** Sage can be very helpful for general hormonal balance during the menopause; and Valerian, Agnus Castus, St John's Wort and Hibiscus are all good for general calming and anxiety. Some herbal manufacturers market a menopause support mix, which combines a number of herbs; again these are available online and in many health food shops. As with all herbal remedies, please check for medication interactions.

- **Supplements.** Magnesium is very good for menopause generally. If you are low on magnesium, as many women are, you are liable to feel anxious. It is naturally calming and helps with anxiety, irritability and mood-changes.

Having mood-swings; feeling down, weepy or angry

Women often experience these feelings due to the menopause, and don't always realise they don't have to.

If you have experienced PMT throughout your life, you might find this is a time when it feels like it is really hitting you and sweeping into your life a whole lot more. Again this is because of the hormonal imbalances of oestrogen and progesterone.

PMT is most likely to occur three to four days before the bleed begins, when the oestrogen is at its lowest and progesterone is building strongly. Classic symptoms are feeling angry or weepy, or sometimes both together, or feeling oversensitive.

During menopause, when the cycle becomes erratic, the hormonal imbalances can cause emotional symptoms similar to PMT, but more extreme or more frequent. Instead of being cyclical (as during the menstrual cycle), oestrogen can be randomly low, and progesterone top heavy in the system. This can occur at any time; and for some women it feels like all the time!

Big mood-swings can have a huge impact on you and your family. You can feel out of control, guilty, and upset because you're not enjoying your friends and family. It can actually seem that you are turning into a bit of dragon – and it's not a nice feeling.

Worse still, you know you are doing it, you can see the results of it, but you feel you can't stop it, so you just carry on. It all feels out of control, and spiralling downwards.

These symptoms are not a normal or inevitable part of menopause at all. It is a sign that there is more imbalance than there need be or is healthy. This is fixable.

So, it's all just down to hormones?

Well, to be frank, not always! The dips and changes in hormones can sometimes have a bit of a 'truth drug' effect. Let's illustrate this with a simple example from one of our clients.

CASE STUDY – BRENDA

'I have always found my in-laws to be a pain in the posterior, but now I find it almost impossible to hide what I feel and still be polite to them. My husband has always been their "little boy" – even though he's now 55!

I've never been good enough. My cooking isn't like my mother-in-law's, my home isn't clean enough, etc. Last Xmas I was going through a really tough time. I was told not to be so selfish; that I was ruining Christmas for my husband and the family, and I should just smile and stop annoying everyone with my problems. Recently I know I've been up and down with moods, but the anger toward my in-laws just bubbles out. I've known them for 30 years; why has it now become so bad? Has menopause really made me so intolerant?'

For Brenda, her anger had a basis, which she had previously kept under wraps. In the past she would have put up with the onslaught from the in-laws until they had left, then opened a bottle of wine and vented for a couple of hours before pushing all the resentment back down again. It had never gone away; she had just suppressed it and seethed quietly between visits. Even her husband didn't realise how humiliated and abused his parents made her feel; he just thought they didn't see eye to eye.

In clinic, we found that the depth of Brenda's negative feelings toward her in-laws went right back to having been made to feel inadequate in childhood, and bullied at school. Her in-laws brought out all these deep feelings in her. During our fertile years, we have normal levels of oestrogen, which is a 'make people happy' hormone, so this had helped Brenda to tuck away all those unhappy feelings of not being good enough – but she had never resolved them. They had now come to the fore, as oestrogen was no longer masking the issue. Her real, deep anger was harder to tuck away, and the truth emerged: that she was fed up with being bullied and put down.

CASE STUDY – BRENDA (FOLLOW UP)

'I am glad I actually looked for some help in the end. Homeopathic counselling really shifted some stuff. It seemed to go back and get to the core of things. For so long, I hadn't really thought about the put-downs and bullying from my childhood. Things improved so quickly after I was treated. I noticed that when my mother-in-law started on me, I could calmly answer her and stand my ground. Things washed over me – I didn't have to try. Sometimes when she came, I just went shopping; I left her with my husband, and I didn't feel guilty! My husband says I am normal again. To be honest, I just feel like myself, act like myself and speak for myself – and it feels great!'

Are my negative feelings a reflection of something deeper?

Negative feelings experienced during the menopause aren't always rooted in childhood experiences, like Brenda's, but there is often a basis to them that ought to be explored. Take some time to really think about what has been happening in your life. Hormonal imbalances can sometimes just 'lower the barrier', so that underlying emotions emerge more easily, and in an uncontrolled way. So if you feel taken for granted, unappreciated or stuck in your life, it might simply be that long-suppressed emotions are now finally coming the surface.

It is important to realise that your feelings are not being created from nothing. If low mood, anger or mood-swings don't settle, it can be very helpful to explore any possible underlying issues. You might find that talking things over with a close and supportive friend is sufficient, or you might decide that you need to consult an experienced homeopathic practitioner or counsellor.

The hormonal changes that happen at this time can act as a catalyst, allowing you really to be yourself and find peace and balance in your life. You might find that you experience a calming effect, or you might see it as an opportunity to make dramatic changes and address things you now realise you have been putting up with. If you follow the clues your body and emotions are giving you, this will help you to find the next piece of the jigsaw-puzzle that is your future.

What treatments can I try?

The following can all help to address negative feelings brought on by the menopause:

- **Homeopathic remedies.** The most effective remedy to try initially is Sepia 200c or 1M. This is a complete hormone balancer. You can buy this online from the homeopathic pharmacies. The other remedy most commonly used for mood-swings is Cimicifuga 1M. This is indicated where you feel under a huge black cloud. Carcinosin 1M is also very useful for balancing hormones, especially if you are feeling overwhelmed. Staphysagria 1M is very good for anger and frustration, to help you find your inner voice. If none of these works for you, you could consider contacting a professional homeopath, as you might need a stronger potency or a different remedy, which they will be able to prescribe.

- **Herbal remedies.** Agnus Castus can be very helpful and balancing to hormones. St John's Wort is good for low mood. As with all herbal remedies, you should discuss with your healthcare provider before using these, to avoid interaction with other medications.

- **Bach Flower Remedies.** Holly can be useful if you are feeling angry and spiteful; Gorse if you are feeling very down and unable to cope.

- **Supplements.** Evening Primrose oil, Star Flower oil and Omega 3 can be helpful. You should always source these from a good company, as cheaper oils might contain contaminants, and you might not get the benefit from them. Taking a high-level Vitamin B supplement can also be useful. Vitamin B6 is good for mood-swings, as it controls hormone production in the brain. There is a natural tendency for Vitamin B to drop around menopause, so supplementing it helps the metabolic process.

- Magnesium oil is known as 'the elixir of youth' – although this might be a little hopeful! It is known that women with PMT symptoms are often low in magnesium, so supplementing it can be useful. High levels of magnesium are needed for hormone production – which is why you might crave dark chocolate! It best absorbed through the skin, so buying a good quality Magnesium oil and rubbing it into a blood-rich area of the body will enable it to be used properly.

Take time to explore what you really feel. If mood-swings and held emotions continue after taking natural remedies it might be worth investigating whether or not there are deeper-rooted feelings that need to be looked into.

And sleep can change too!

A change in sleep pattern is an incredibly common symptom of menopause, and this is something that is frequently overlooked. It is often attributed instead to stress, or diet, or getting older. If a connection to the menopause is made, it is often simplified as hot flushes disturbing the sleep. While physical symptoms such as hot flushes can indeed disturb the sleep, that isn't the whole story, and the disruption can continue long after hot flushes have ceased. In our clinic we have met many women worried that they are suffering disruption to their sleep pattern, and who haven't realised that this can often be due to the hormonal changes of the menopause.

It is really useful to understand that sleep doesn't naturally come in a solid eight-hour block. A lot of people believe that they need this eight-hour block, otherwise they will become unwell. Actually, sleep is made up of small blocks of approximately one and a half to two hours each. These are called sleep cycles.

In one sleep cycle, you will experience all the different phases of sleep, including light sleep, deep sleep and dream sleep. These are all important for maintaining physical wellbeing, cell renewal, emotional health, including memory, and general psychological wellbeing.

At the end of each sleep cycle, the body naturally goes into a very light sleep, almost awake, then drifts back into another sleep cycle. This gives the impression of a continuous period of sleep. So eight hours' sleep is really made up of four or more separate sleep cycles!

When your body is almost awake, which is at the end of a natural sleep cycle, it is easy for it to become fully awake. So, for example, if you need to go the loo, or if you are preoccupied by everyday ongoing worries, this will be the time when you wake up. Normally it is relatively easy to drop back to sleep, because this has followed a natural break and there is a natural start to a new sleep cycle.

At menopause it is not uncommon for this sleep pattern to change. Either the sleep cycles become shorter, or the way they flow into each other changes, so that one or even two complete cycles are, in effect, missed out.

The most common pattern described to us by menopausal women in our clinic is that they have two full sleep cycles, then miss a cycle (stay awake for one and a half to two hours), then one more sleep cycle, then another period of wakefulness (which might be shorter) and then another full sleep cycle.

So, if you go to bed at 10.00 pm, you might find that you wake at 2.00 am; stay awake until 4.00 am; sleep again until 6.00 am; are then briefly awake; and lastly go back to sleep until 8.00 am. Unfortunately, for many women in this position, sleeping until 8.00 am doesn't fit with their normal working hours or family commitments, so they end up feeling sleep-deprived and anxious that nothing seems to be helping.

CASE STUDY – JOANNE

Joanne came to see us with symptoms of digestive problems and sleep disturbance. Previously she had always been a great sleeper, getting eight to ten hours every night without any difficulty. Now she said she was getting three to four hours at most. She was unable to function at work and was getting grumpy with her husband.

After homeopathic treatment, she felt better, but still thought she wasn't sleeping properly. After talking through her sleep diary with us, she realised that she was actually getting a four hour block of sleep; one hour awake; two hours of sleep; half an hour awake; and one and a half hours of sleep. So, while this was different from her usual pattern, she was getting more sleep that she had realised. No wonder she was feeling better! It really relieved her anxiety to understand the cyclical pattern.

Many people recognise that melatonin is an important sleep hormone, and plays a vital role in us falling asleep and staying asleep. It is the hormone that is disrupted by jetlag and shift working. It is known to interact with other female hormones such as luteinising hormone and progesterone. So it is easy to see why the hormonal changes occurring during the menopause will affect sleep. Balancing your hormones across the board will help to improve things generally – including your sleep pattern.

So, what can I do to help myself sleep better?

First of all, you need to get your hormones properly balanced. Are the hot flushes disturbing you at night? If this is the major cause of lack of sleep, have a look through Chapter Four and the advice on managing hot flushes.

If you are feeling unsettled or worried in your life, especially with the mood-swings and anxiety that can accompany the menopause, this too can disturb your sleep. Have a look at the earlier parts of this chapter to address this.

Other helpful approaches are:

- **Keep a sleep diary.** It could be that, like our client Joanne, you are getting more sleep than you think, but simply not in the pattern that you used to. It might help you to understand how long your sleep cycles are, and not become anxious at waking.

- **Practise relaxation and meditation.** Yes, this really can help. It can be annoying to be told to relax when you feel stressed, but it is worth trying. If you don't naturally find it easy, there are many useful apps that have relaxation recordings.

- **Burning essential oils can be very restful.** There are many available, and lots of helpful books about them. Lavender can be used, either as an essential oil or on the pillow;

and there are even specialist lavender pillows that can be bought. Adding four to six drops of an essential oil to your bath water can be very relaxing. Alternatively you can add drops of an essential oil into a carrier oil such as coconut oil or almond oil (commonly 15 drops of essential oil to 500ml of carrier oil) and massage it into your skin before sleep. Explore what works best for you. Never apply neat essential oil to the skin; always dilute, and skin test first.

• **Herbal remedies.** Those containing Valerian and Hops can be helpful. Some companies market over-the-counter combinations that naturally promote relaxation and help you to drift off to sleep more easily. Kalms is one example. These are worth trying, though some will probably work better for you than others.

• **Homeopathic remedies**. Passiflora can help, and some homeopathic pharmacies produce combination remedies e.g. Helios Sleep. Copper Beech can also be effective; and, again, try Nux Vomica if you are feeling anxious.

• **Bach Flower Remedies**. White Chestnut is good for recurrent thoughts that stop sleeping.

• **Common sense!** Avoiding staring at computer screens or watching scary movies just before bed. Ensure that your bedroom is comfortable, cool and dark, and that you have the right number of covers on your bed – it is easy to become overheated at this time, even if hot flushes aren't especially an issue. Avoid stimulating drinks containing caffeine for a few hours before sleep.

Summary

Emotional symptoms, such as anxiety and mood-swings, can be just as disruptive as the more commonly recognised physical symptoms of the menopause. They can be entirely caused by hormonal disturbances, or partly influenced by them. So take control of finding help for yourself rather than just feel down or guilty.

Emotional symptoms might come without physical symptoms – so don't just dismiss them as being not part of the menopause simply because you don't see anything else, such as hot flushes, going on at the same time.

Some emotional symptoms such as anger or feeling unappreciated can have deeper roots. So if you think this might be the case, and you might perhaps have been previously suppressing your true emotions, take the time now to try to access them and get to the root of the problem.

Sleep often changes with menopause. Take some time to learn about your sleep pattern and experiment with natural remedies to see what helps most of all.

6 HOW DO I STOP MY BONES GETTING WEAK?

I want to make sure that my bones are okay – what can I do?

When they are younger, most women don't even think about how strong or weak their bones are. The onset of menopausal symptoms can often be the prompt for this to become an issue, and for them to start to worry that their bones are beginning to fade away – rapidly!

In fact, their bones will have been ageing and changing for many years, in some cases even decades, prior to the menopause – but usually without any signs or symptoms.

CASE STUDY – EILEEN

'I was in the chemist's and they were offering bone density scans. My friend wanted one done, so I went along with it too. I was only 40, so it was really only out of curiosity. I wasn't in the least bit worried or even interested. The big shock was, even though she was ten years older than me, her results were great, whereas mine were shocking! I had a bone age of 55! It was such a wake-up call. I realised I had been taking this for granted – why wouldn't it be fine? I'd had no intention of even thinking about it until I was very old (perhaps 50!) I'd thought I was active, but really I probably spent more time in the car running the

kids to their after-school stuff. I started yoga and pilates, and realised just how unfit I had become. Somehow I had thought that my 30-year-old body would just kind of carry on.'

There are a lot of factors that can exacerbate bone loss, including poor diet, lack of exercise and some medication side-effects – all of which precede the better-known downturn of oestrogen that occurs at menopause. So beginning to look after our bones as soon as possible in life, and entering our middle years with the best possible start, is important and really makes a difference.

It is important to realise that bones are not simply solid sticks providing scaffolding to the muscles and the flesh. They are very complex structures that are constantly rebuilding, growing and changing – and providing all sorts of useful things for the body. They produce blood cells and platelets; they store minerals; they regulate the acid base balance in the body; and they are vital to the immune system.

Generally keeping fit and well, with good exercise and diet, is vital for every aspect of health. However, extra considerations arise at the menopause; and there are steps you can take that will make a difference and keep your bones strong and active as you age.

What happens at menopause that changes normal bone strength?

A complex, dense matrix of calcium, collagen and other key minerals wraps itself around cells known as osteoblasts and hardens to form bones. As with all cells in the body, these grow, die and regenerate throughout life.

Oestrogen has a protective effect on bones, and although it is not really understood how this works, it is clear that unless the changes that occur at menopause are carefully managed, this can have a negative impact on bone strength and increase your risk of fractures as you get older. The big problem is that this symptom might not be obvious. Unless you have a bone density scan – or worse, an accident – you might be completely unaware of the state of your bone health.

While the full interactions aren't completely understood, some of the mechanisms are. One of the more recent ideas is that oestrogen acts to reduce the effect of an enzyme – caspase-3 – that is known to be responsible for initiating the loss of osteoblasts i.e. the bone-building cells.[2] If this is so, it means that normal levels of oestrogen in pre-menopausal women act to restrain the destructive effect of caspase-3. In short, oestrogen keeps the destruction at bay. So, at menopause, when the overall oestrogen level drops, or becomes chaotic, the enzyme has more free rein.

However, this is only one aspect of a complete hormonal, physiological and mechanical picture – especially taking into account that the bones might have become thinner long before any change in oestrogen at peri-menopause or menopause.

Is hormone replacement therapy (HRT) the answer?

It is too simplistic to think that a loss of bone strength stemming from the downturn in overall oestrogen levels at the menopause

---

[2] *Bradford et al 2007.*

can be addressed just by adding in synthetic oestrogen in the form of medication. Simply taking HRT that includes oestrogen is a one-sided approach to a more complex, holistic issue.

We have a deep culture in the Western world of expecting 'a pill for every ill'. This can lead to a passive approach of looking outside of ourselves for something or someone else to fix our problems. Especially when science suggests a link between losing a particular chemical and synthetically replacing it with a tablet, many people feel that this counts as restoring a normal balance. Sadly this doesn't reflect this reality of all the steps necessary for women to maintain their health and wellbeing.

Again, prevention is better than cure. Natural ageing does have effects on the body, but although you can't reverse it, you can reverse or prevent many age-related problems. You can start yoga and ballet when you are 55! Pre-empting a problem at the start of peri-menopause, or at age 50 or even older, is much better than leaving it until becomes life-restricting.

What can I do to help myself and my bones?

There is a great deal that you as an individual can do to influence your general bone health at this time, and indeed at any time in your life. Actually using your bones – i.e. taking exercise – has been shown to be particularly useful in this regard. It also has wider benefits. In one study[3], regular physical activity was found to substantially improve sleep, reduce anxiety, help with hot flushes and improve sexual health. This demonstrates the real health risks posed by our increasingly sedentary lifestyle. However, it is also

---

[3] *Mansikkamaki et al 2014*

encouraging, as it means that we can make lifestyle changes to reduce those risks. It is not reasonable to expect a drug solution to something that can be easily improved by lifestyle changes.

What exercises would help my bones?

Weight-bearing exercises help keep bones strong by causing the muscles and tendons to pull on them – stimulating the bone cells to produce more bone. This is the easiest kind of exercise to incorporate into your life if you aren't really a gym bunny and don't have a current exercise regime such as jogging. It uses your own body weight to create the stress and promote the growth of bone.

Simple exercise:

- **Walking.** Walking for a couple of hours a day has been shown to reduce hip fractures and improve bone health in women of post-menopausal age. Even if you can't manage two hours at a time, shorter walks are still worth doing. Be active.

- **Balancing.** Balancing on one leg for a time loads more of your body weight onto the bones than they usually carry. Leaning forward with your palms against a wall and your arms supporting your weight achieves the same for those bones. This can really improve both bone strength and muscle tone. The advantage of the balancing approach, particularly if you don't have a naturally active life, is that it can be easily added into your daily routine – e.g. standing on one leg while waiting for the kettle to boil, or waiting at the photocopier at work, or cleaning your teeth. In fact, at any time when you are standing, as long as you are well balanced and upright, you can use one leg instead of two. Make sure you don't topple over though!

• **Yoga.** Yoga doesn't stress cartilage or joints; instead it lengthens the muscles and holds them there, creating tension in the bone. Well-known postures such as the 'plank' – which puts pressure on the arms and feet – or the 'warrior' – which puts pressure on the legs, hips and shoulders – or a sequence such as the 'sun salutation' – which stretches and exercises muscles and joints – are all beneficial to bone health. There are many other useful postures; and if you aren't familiar with yoga, taking classes is a great way of strengthening bones, as well as muscles and tendons, to keep the body both supple and strong.

More advanced exercise:

Adding impact into weight-bearing exercise has been shown to be incredibly beneficial to bone health; and sudden impact or shock to the bone increases the rate of new bone build.

• **Jogging.** Although it uses only the body's own weight, the extra benefit of impact when jogging or running is noticeable. Before you begin, make sure you have professionally-fitted running shoes; a good professional should be able to match your individual form and gait with specialist shoes that will help to ensure you don't get injuries. Many local authorities have low-cost running groups for beginners who would like help starting out. For the more advanced, or those seeking support and advice, gyms and running clubs abound, and are always keen for new members.

- **Bouncing.** Yes, bouncing on a trampoline (or mini trampoline at home) is another excellent way to strengthen your bones!

- **Gym.** The use of dumbbells and multi-gym machines increases the weight impact-to-exercise ratio and therefore helps build healthy bones.

- The key thing with exercise is to pick something that you like doing and can incorporate readily into your life. Perhaps there is a sport that you previously enjoyed and that you can return to. Make sure you find the type of exercise that works for you, and do it regularly. Don't set yourself up to fail.

Diet

One of the very first things that women at the onset of menopause often say to us – even before mentioning hot flushes or other symptoms – is that they feel they must increase their calcium intake or start taking calcium supplements, as they are worried about their bone health. However, this is based on a misconception.

Calcium and Vitamin D

Contrary to popular belief, with a normal broad, healthy diet, we are nowadays very unlikely to have insufficient calcium in the food we eat. The difficulty actually comes in absorbing the calcium. Our bodies need Vitamin D in order to be able to do this, and it is extremely common to be Vitamin D-deficient.

Very few foods contain Vitamin D; instead, it is produced mainly by the exposure of our skin to the sun. As well as having long, dark winters and cloudy summer days that reduce such exposure, we tend to spend a lot of our lives indoors. Even if out in the sun, we generally cover up with clothes or sunscreen. In a stark illustration of this point, a recent study has shown that over one third of Australians are Vitamin D-deficient. [4] Although living in one of the world's sunniest countries, they block the sun from reaching their skin, impacting their health. Such caution is perhaps understandable, given the very reasonable fears about skin cancer; but it is all a question of balance.

Many studies have been carried out in Finland where, due to its geographical location in Northern Europe and consequent shortage of sunlight, the authorities are extremely interested in the role of Vitamin D in the body. They have found that historical recommendations on the ideal level of Vitamin D have been too low.

So, increasing our Vitamin D intake is a really positive step we can take in order to increase our calcium absorption, improve our bone density and strengthen our muscle fibres. It has also been shown to have tentative links to other health benefits such as, for children, reducing the risk of developing Type 1 diabetes. Some research has also linked Vitamin D deficiency to pathological inflammatory bowel disease and colon cancer. All in all, it is a very important vitamin.

Other supplements

Vitamin E, Vitamin K, magnesium and boron are also good to

---

[4] *http://www.deakin.edu.au/research/stories/2012/01/16/ vitamin-d-deficiency-strikes-one-third-of-australians*

take for bone strength. You can buy these as a combination mix. However, it is important to note that quality really matters here. The problem with supplements is that they can be difficult for the body to break down. Cheaper, poor-quality products are not fully absorbed, so you will not reap the benefit that you might expect from them. We recommend good-quality food-state supplements. Although they are often a little more expensive to buy, you will be absorbing and using more of them and getting the maximum health benefits, and therefore ultimately better value for money.

Alkali-forming foods are better for maintaining good bones

A typical western European diet is very high in acid-forming foods. This doesn't actually relate to whether the foods are acid or alkaline in themselves, but to how they are metabolised within the body. Acid-forming foods include meat, white rice, white bread, fats, processed foods, fizzy drinks, sugar, coffee and most simple carbohydrates.

To ensure the body's systems function properly, it is critical for it to maintain at all costs a stable pH balance – that is, a stable acid-alkali balance. If there are high levels of acid-forming foods in the diet, the acid has to be neutralised; and if there is no other source of alkali, the body will do this by stripping alkaline minerals from itself. Calcium is one such mineral, and might be stripped from the bone. To prevent this happening, it is therefore important to ensure that sufficient alkali-forming foods are consumed.

Good alkali-forming foods include nearly all fruit and vegetables, brown rice, quinoa, almonds and cold pressed oils such as olive oil.

Simply changing the balance of your diet can be extremely beneficial to your bone health – and also have the positive side-effect of helping you to maintain a healthy weight.

Phyto-oestrogens for bones

A lot has been written about phyto-oestrogens, and the debate rages on, with at times conflicting evidence on their benefits and disbenefits.

Menopausal clients commonly come to us with the belief that, as their own oestrogen level is dropping, they need to increase the intake of phyto-oestrogens in their diet. However, the situation isn't really that clear-cut. As explained in Chapter One, the oestrogen level doesn't simply drop during the menopause. Rather, it becomes highly variable, and does not finally drop until after the menopause is complete. Plus, the body can obtain oestrogen from sources other than the well-known one of the ovaries.

Having said this, while the evidence is still not as clear as we would wish, there is some indication that taking phyto-oestrogens is beneficial. Some women have reported reduced hot flushes, improved bone health and improved cardiovascular health. There could also be a link to reduced breast cancer risk, although this last claimed benefit is not at all certain.

More research is ideally needed on this; but unfortunately it seems highly unlikely that there will ever be sufficiently large trials carried out to build a conclusive evidence base. Large trials are extremely expensive, and funding them is often a problem. At present, most medical research is undertaken by large pharmaceutical companies, who aim to recoup their investment by marketing a resulting drug. If the appropriate treatment would be not a drug but instead a readily-available natural substance, there is no economic case for investing in trials.

Examples of foods containing phyto-oestrogens are fermented soya, hops, dandelion, red clover, sage, alfalfa and flaxseeds.

Summary

Taking care of your bones is not just a menopausal issue, but important to all aspects of your health, and should be thought about throughout your life, not just as you get older.

Exercise and diet really do make a difference. Take time to study how much exercise you have and what your diet is actually like, rather than assume you are probably doing okay.

Find a type of exercise that works for you and fits your routine – even taking some time each day to balance on one leg will help improve your bone strength.

Make simple changes to your diet that you can manage and enjoy. You will feel better if you find a diet that improves your bones and general health; eating food that you hate, just because it is 'healthy', will not necessarily be of any benefit to you, and you won't stick to it.

Eat less processed and acid-forming food, and reduce your sugar intake.

Take control. It's never too late to make positive changes!

7 I AM SCARED ABOUT MENOPAUSE

'I don't want to have strange symptoms and become asexual. Actually, I dread that I might feel less of a woman.'

There are a lot of negative stereotypes about ageing that pervade our society. The media is chock-a-block with the horrors of the menopause and all the symptoms we are supposed to experience. As well as sounding fairly unpleasant, these symptoms are connected to the idea of becoming an 'old hag', losing self-image and personality and becoming someone new, who is now the opposite of young and attractive.

A great deal of imagery that pervades our society connects youth with attractiveness and sexuality, while older women are connected with being unattractive and worn out. We are in a culture that is a youth-obsessed. Older women can feel invisible – and the menopause can mark this change, making it more apparent. In fact, 'menopausal' has often been colloquially used as a term to describe an older, stubborn, difficult woman. Why wouldn't any woman feel scared to face this?

This is a state of affairs that is wrong at every level. The image needs to be updated and changed to reflect the reality. Menopause is a time of freedom to be embraced, a time of wisdom to be enjoyed and a time of self-discovery to be cherished.

This chapter explains the process and the possibilities, and gives tips to overcome common problems.

This is a time of change

Some women are extremely frightened by what is seemingly the impending doom that is menopause. Other are less so, approaching it more with a feeling of a curiosity and wonder as to what it will mean for them. But even if you are one of those who are feeling relatively positive about menopause, you are bound to find it a time of change. For most people, change that comes about not of their own choosing – and without their permission! – is difficult. You don't know how this is going to be for you, what symptoms you might or might not have, or how severe they might be. You don't know how long it is going to last. You don't necessarily know what to do for the best.

CASE STUDY – YVONNE

'I was just waltzing toward the menopause, thinking it would be just fine. Quite looking forward to my periods stopping, because they were just annoying. They became a bit more erratic, which was fine – and then I had my first real hot flushes. Oh my God, I wasn't expecting that! I realised that I was totally unprepared, and I had been completely ignoring what it might mean for me. I'd assumed that I would be able to carry on as before but just not have periods, which didn't seem so bad. I took a real about-turn, and realised that actually I was ageing, and my sex drive and response were changing. Surprisingly I was worried about getting old and not being attractive. Somehow I'd thought it would all happen "over there" and I would stay pretty much the

same; but it was me this was happening to. I was having to cope with real changes. At first I was scared, but I realised I had to face this and see where it might lead.'

\\

Yvonne is typical of many women who have balanced hormones and are really just bored with having a cycle. They are surprised by how many different and unexpected feelings the menopause brings up. For example, they might suddenly feel fearful or grief-stricken at the thought of being unable to have any more children, even though their family is grown up and they don't actually want any more. It doesn't always seem to make sense; but this is all about a loss of opportunity, choice and control.

Things are changing, and you have little choice about the fact this is happening. However, you have a lot of choice about how you approach the experience, and thrive through it.

This book has chapters dedicated to other aspects of menopause, but one of the least discussed is how it can affect a woman's sexuality.

Will I lose my sex drive?

In short, no! Although there is a hormonal basis to women's sex drive, it is only one aspect of the whole picture. Let's look at that picture.

During a normal ovulatory cycle prior to the menopause, a woman's libido or sex drive will tend to rise in the few days preceding ovulation, which usually occurs about mid-cycle. So, for women with a 28-day cycle, the libido will usually rise on about day 11 through to day 14. For those with a longer cycle – say, 32 days – ovulation might occur a little later, perhaps on day 18, and the libido will usually rise on about day 14 through to day 18.

This has a biological basis: having a higher sex drive at the time when she will be producing an egg increases a woman's chance of conceiving. However, as all women know, these three or four days of the month are not the only time when sexual urges can arise! This shows that oestrogen, and oestrogen surges, are only one factor.

While still having a menstrual cycle – indicating a natural rise and fall of oestrogen – women will report having a particular normal level of sex drive. For some it is high; they have strong urges most of the time, and these become even stronger with the oestrogen surge just before ovulation. Others have no strong urges; they are perhaps ambivalent for most of the month, but can feel a slight rise in interest just before ovulation. Most women fall somewhere between these two ends of the spectrum. Our natural level of sex drive is something that is individual to each of us. You will probably recognise your own.

So, in short, sex drive does not disappear at menopause. You will continue to have your own natural level, with shifts caused by more random oestrogen surges. The variability is key here. Oestrogen does not disappear from the body; menopause causes a change in where and how it is produced. Instead of it being produced from the ovaries, it is produced from the adrenal glands and fatty tissues. So, even when menopausal, we are still sexual beings – if we choose to be, of course!

Discovering your natural sex drive

Women who have a healthy and balanced menopause should find that their natural sex drive returns after the onset of menopause. If it doesn't, this is a sign that there is some other issue – physical, hormonal or emotional – that needs to be addressed!

If you feel you might be in this position, it is worth first of all considering the following:

- If you still have a cycle, how does your libido change during the month? If it is normally quite flat for most of the time, with a slight increase only shortly before ovulation, it could be that you are just one of those women (and men) who naturally have a lower sex drive.

- Are there some days or times – when you are relaxed or on holiday, for instance – when your sex drive feels higher? If this is the case, your sex drive is still there, but might need some help to return to its normal level.

What if I think things aren't how they should be?

Losing libido and becoming asexual are not a necessary consequence of the menopause itself. Sex drive can be affected by other issues such as mood, personal confidence, body confidence, and the emotional connection you feel to yourself as well as to your partner.

Case Study – Hannah

'I have such a lovely husband. We have been married for 30 years, and he is kind and understanding, which makes me feel even worse. I just don't feel like having sex at all. He is a lovely guy who still fancies me, and I feel like I keep making excuses and backing away. He's been really understanding, but I feel bad.

'I came for treatment with Anne and Claire because my hot flushes and mood-swings were dreadful. These symptoms cleared up immediately, which was great, but I still didn't feel like having sex. I realised that although my hormones were now fine, this hadn't improved my sex drive.

'After careful counselling and analysis with Anne and Claire, it became clear that my problem wasn't actually menopause-related. I'd always had weight issues – I've been on every diet known to man – and to be honest I really hated my body. I actually found it disgusting! I realised that this was really standing in the way. No matter how often my husband told me I was beautiful, it didn't matter.

'Anne and Claire gave me some hypnotherapy, which removed my deep fear of ageing and disgust at my body. This completely changed everything. Now both my hormones and my mind are balanced, and things with my husband are the best they've ever been. With the children leaving home, we now have the time to enjoy things too!'

Body image is an important factor, especially as we age. Our mind remains young, but in the mirror we see our body looking different from how we feel it should. If – as with Hannah – this has always been a worry, even when youth was on our side, it is worth taking time to get to the root of the problem. There are lots of ways to approach this.

Finding holistic body confidence

Some women have found it a useful self-help approach to learn to love and accept their body by experiencing and appreciating how it feels when it moves and functions. Both physical and mental freedom can be found by allowing the body and mind to work together in activities such as:

- sport (e.g. running, cycling, badminton);

- something more spiritual (e.g. yoga, meditation, pilates); or

- something creative (e.g. dance).

This takes the body into being just one part of who we are holistically; a tool to express our true inner self. We are more than just a set of vital statistics.

Self-image – seeing yourself

Many women who visit our clinic have an uneasy relationship with their body and their sexuality. They might feel that this has been caused by a particular life event (such as childbirth), or has arisen only with the onset of menopause and ageing. Often, however, seeing themselves as a confident sexual being, and enjoying themselves openly with a partner, has actually been a big deal for them throughout their lives, and has only got worse at this time. Underlying issues with confidence and sexuality might simply have been less apparent prior to the menopause, because the oestrogen surges that occur around ovulation can be strong enough to override insecurities and allow a more healthy sex life.

Part of the work we do in our clinic is with women who have difficulties with their self-image. Ideas of what is a good or 'perfect' physical look have changed constantly over history – but they have always been around. Trying to conform to what is a shifting and unreliable ideal will always be unsuccessful. With the routine use of photo-manipulation software these days, so many images that are presented as ideal are actually fake, and it's no wonder we can feel inadequate.

Self-image is about more than what you see in the mirror, or how your appearance compares with other people's. It is about how you feel about yourself.

Sometimes your confidence can falter for simple reasons. You might have lost the motivation to maintain your health or fitness; you might have lost touch with friends who kept you feeling connected and happy; or you might have lost the time and energy to keep up with hobbies that made you feel good.

For example, you might have liked playing badminton or tennis, but then got out of the habit, without realising that it gave you a sense of wellbeing and confidence and made you feel positive about yourself. Or perhaps you used to have regular lunches with friends and go shopping with them afterwards –

buying clothes or make-up and finding fun in looking after yourself and trying new fashions and ideas. Finding time to re-establish these former routines, and keeping things light and fun, can often help.

However, much more often, poor self-image can arise from deeper issues. The most common of these we encounter in our clinic are childhood trauma; abuse; eating disorders from adolescence; yo-yo dieting; unrealistic expectations of what constitutes 'the perfect body'; and fear of growing older. Working through these issues, and helping people to break through the negative perceptions and find a sense of self and personal power, brings real and permanent improvements.

If you feel there is something from your younger life that might be affecting you now, and that might stop you making the important transition of menopause successfully and positively, now is the time to address it. Here are some possible approaches:

- **Counselling**. This can be very useful, but be sure you find a counsellor with whom you have good connection – don't just stick with someone who doesn't feel right.

- **Homeopathic counselling**. This is a targeted, solution-based counselling system supported by homeopathic remedies to maximise the speed of recovery.

- **Hypnotherapy**. This is an excellent way of tapping into unconscious fears and anxieties and can be very successful. Again, make sure you are comfortable with the therapist before beginning treatment, and don't stick with someone if things don't feel right.

- **Homeopathy.** A good homeopathic practitioner who is experienced in dealing with deeper emotional issues can help to find remedies that will move this along quickly. This approach can used alongside counselling and hypnotherapy.

- **EFT (Emotional Freedom Technique).** This involves tapping on key acupressure points on the body, and can help to eradicate negative thought-patterns. A good book to read if you want to learn more about how you can help yourself with this technique is Isy Grigg's EFT in Your Pocket (New Vision Media, 2005).

- **Yoga.** This is excellent for developing confidence and learning to move the body in new ways, developing strength and flexibility. It releases trapped emotions from parts of the body that might be particularly holding fear and negativity.

- **Mindfulness meditation.** This develops the ability to find peace and to silence the internal critic, so that you can develop kindness toward yourself.

What else might the problem be if my libido feels unnaturally low?

Another possible cause of low libido is using hormonal contraceptives. The pill, the hormonal coil and the implant are all intended to disrupt your normal cycle, lowering the hormone levels so that you do not ovulate and therefore do not get pregnant. It is not at all surprising for women to have a much reduced libido if they are using hormonal contraceptives. For some, this effect persists even after they have come off the contraceptives. When we find this issue with clients in our clinic, we treat it homeopathically; but other natural treatments such as acupuncture or herbs can be very effective too. Typical treatments are:

- **Homeopathic:** Sepia 200, Folliculinum 200.

- **Herbal:** Agnus Castus.

Grief and shock can also lead to reduced libido, along with other profound effects on the body and emotions. They can cause the brain to produce chemicals that trigger a cascade effect, suppressing natural sex hormones.

Even if the loss or shock happened some time ago, or was not unexpected (e.g. a death after a long illness), that doesn't mean that you should just 'get over it' and forget about it. Recognise that this is okay. Time doesn't always heal, although people will probably tell you that it does. You might well need to get help and support. If you haven't felt well ever since a particular incident or event took place, don't just wait for this to go away; it might actually get worse.

Homeopathic remedies that can be useful here are Ignatia 1M (for grief) and Aconite 1M (for shock).

In brief, if you feel your libido has dipped, ask yourself:

- Could this have been caused by using hormonal contraceptives? These can massively suppress your sex drive – and it doesn't necessarily return once you stop using them.

- How do you feel about your appearance? If you have deep-rooted body-image issues, you might need professional help to overcome them; but sometimes just trying some type of regular physical activity, such as dancing or a sport, can make a big difference.

- Has the change in your libido coincided with a change of partner? If your current partner is making you feel bad, you might want to consider if he or she is the right one for you!

- Has your sex drive changed since childbirth? This could be either a hormonal or a psychological issue, as your body will have undergone changes; and you might need professional help to address it. If childbirth had a severe physical impact, investigate if there are medical options to improve things. Don't think that the problem will just go away in time, or that there is no point bothering now you are near menopause.

- Have you suffered any major grief or upset from which you don't feel fully recovered?

- Does your libido change when you are on holiday or relaxed?

If one or more of the above points strikes a chord with you, then these wider issues might well underlie the change in your libido or in your self-confidence or self-image. So simply jumping onto the hormone drug approach might not resolve your issue at all.

My libido is fine, but sex is painful. Is this normal?

There is a commonly-held belief that women 'dry up' at menopause. In most cases, this is untrue. There are, though, some important changes that take place, and that you should be prepared for. You might feel less lubricated, and if it does hurt to have intercourse, you ought to keep track of this and have it checked out by a medical professional. The practice nurse at your doctor's surgery will be very used to doing smear tests, and will be able to give you an examination and offer advice if you are worried.

There are a couple of things to look out for in order to ensure that your vagina stays healthy. The first is the health of the vaginal tissues themselves. This is maintained by the same nutritional foundations that help to keep general skin and connective tissues healthy and elastic. Collagen is the main influence, and as we age, its levels drop and the skin becomes thinner and less elastic. Having a good diet and vitamin intake can minimise this effect, although it might still become gradually more noticeable with age.

The second issue is the hormones that produce mucus and therefore lubrication. Prior to the menopause, hormones influence the production of mucus of different types at different times of the menstrual cycle. This natural lubrication comes from glands high up inside the vagina, near the neck of the uterus. It moves slowly down the vagina, removing dead cells, keeping it clean, supple and moist. It is naturally slightly acidic, which helps to prevent infection. This is a constant natural process that helps to keep the vagina healthy.

During menopause, a lot of women notice that the production of mucus gradually reduces, and the general background feeling of lubrication can be lacking. Some women might feel a little dryer. However, it should never be uncomfortable. The experience of 'wetness' or 'dryness' is different for different woman; but by the end of the menopause, all will have lost the cyclical hormonal influence from their regular periods, and ought therefore to take extra care to support their vaginal health.

It is vital that you are vigilant for any signs of discomfort, and do not simply put up with anything that feels 'wrong'. Many women think it is a natural part of menopause that they have to put up with feeling dry, and don't follow up symptoms such as pain, irritation or burning – but this is absolutely not true. You shouldn't even wait until there are problematic symptoms. If things don't feel quite right, have this checked. Your practice nurse will be ideally qualified to advise you.

If you are having regular smear tests, it is always worth asking the medical practitioner who carries these out to check the health of your cervix and vagina. Ask if there are any signs of the tissue looking dry or thin. They will be very happy to chat to you about how things look and, if they are okay now, when they ought to be checked again.

There are a number of things you can do to pre-empt problems, but once the vaginal tissue does become thin, there is very little that can be done retrospectively to improve this. If you are unsure, always ask your practice nurse to check – don't wait.

What can be done to help with vaginal dryness?

Firstly and most importantly – because we can't say it often enough – don't leave it too late. Have regular health checks, and if you are at all worried, seek your medical practitioner's advice. Always ask at any smear test what things look like, and if they are as healthy as they should be. Other helpful steps to take are as follows:

- **Diet**. Make sure you have a really good diet that supports skin health and collagen production. Vitamin C, which is in citrus foods, helps prevent free-radical damage;

Omega 3 particularly helps protect the fatty cells around skin membrane; lycopene protects the skin; green leafy vegetables are rich in antioxidants; and lean proteins are important too.

• **Magnesium supplement.** Magnesium is an excellent supplement to support skin and hormonal balance. It is best absorbed trans-dermally (through the skin), so we would recommend using a good magnesium spray daily, applying it directly to the skin. There are many on the market, and they will have clear directions on how to use them – common advice is to apply about a teaspoon at a time to blood-rich areas of the body (feet, legs etc). The spray usually needs to be left on the body for at least twenty minutes, after which you can wash it off and apply your usual perfume if you wish. These are general instructions only; it is important to check the label of your particular supplier.

• **Oestrogen pessaries.** If the skin inside the vagina is thinning, you should consider taking action to stop this from getting worse. A local oestrogen pessary can be used, on prescription from your doctor. This puts oestrogen directly into the vagina, which helps mucus production and also supports the skin and tissues. It prevents further thinning of the skin, which in turn helps keep the vagina elastic and feeling comfortable.

• **Natural progesterone cream.** Some women use a natural progesterone cream. A very small amount is simply applied to a fat-rich area of the skin, which absorbs it gradually. You should follow the instructions given on your particular brand of cream; these will detail how much to use and how many times a week to suit your individual needs. A general starting point is to use just a pea-sized amount three times a week.

- **Herbs.** Some of the most common herbs found to be potentially helpful are Motherwort (Leonurus Cardiac) or Chaste Tree (Vitex/Agnus Castus). Use ten to twenty drops of the tincture in water two to three times daily or, if bought in tablet form, as directed. Black Cohosh and Wild Yam as herbal supplements are also helpful for some women.

- **Water-based lubricants and vaginal moisturisers.** These can be used to alleviate vaginal dryness and improve general vaginal health.

- **Avoid perfumed products.** Stay away from highly-perfumed soaps and bath products. Be aware, also, that some products marketed as 'natural' aren't really so; you really have to read the labels to check the ingredients! Feminine hygiene products such as scented wipes and washes can interfere with the natural balance of the vagina, and can make you prone to contracting thrush.

Foreplay works!

Both before and after the menopause, sexual arousal normally causes two glands (the Bartholins glands) at the entrance to the vagina to release extra moisture and mucus, which can help in sexual intercourse. In the months leading up to the menopause, there is a decrease in the 'background' level of hormonal mucus that is produced. If sexual arousal is insufficient to cause the Bartholins glands to produce a good amount of moisture, this becomes more noticeable, as the decrease in the 'background' level means that it no longer makes up for any such lack.

Taking more time on foreplay will help, as will avoiding stress and feeling relaxed. Natural lubricants can also be used. Other helpful things to try are dietary changes, magnesium supplements and use of oestrogen cream or pessaries, as outlined above.

Don't forget that, until you have had no bleeds for a complete year, you can still randomly ovulate, and therefore, if you are having unprotected sex, conceive. If pregnancy is really not part of your life plan at this time, you should continue to use contraception.

Once you have completed menopause, your periods have stopped for a year and you are symptom free, it is true that your oestrogen level will begin to settle and drop. Tests on women aged 70 plus show them having levels of oestrogen that are low and stable. At this more settled time, there is no question of experiencing peaks and lows of oestrogen, and still women can have a good sex life and a good sex drive. So there is obviously more to this than just oestrogen and youth – in fact, by this age, you might have picked up a few more tricks!

Summary

Ageing does not mean losing your sexuality. Your libido might shift, but your sex drive does not disappear.

If you notice that your libido is flagging, do not just assume this is a natural part of ageing. Look for life changes, life events or deeper emotional scars that might have been acquired during your life, and if necessary obtain external help.

Good quality hypnotherapy, counselling, homeopathy, homeopathic counselling, mindfulness meditation and yoga can all be very helpful in working through mental and emotional challenges. Simple lifestyle changes, such as connecting with friends and pursuing hobbies, can be very helpful too.

Look after your vaginal health. Do not accept dryness or discomfort. Steps such as dietary changes, taking herbal supplements, vitamins and mineral supplements, and using oestrogen cream or pessaries, can prevent permanent damage occurring.

Foreplay works, so enjoy.

8   IS HORMONE REPLACEMENT THERAPY (HRT) A GOOD OPTION?

I'm confused: is HRT a problem or a potential solution?

Since the 1970s, HRT has been commonly prescribed as a first-line therapy. To start with, it was often offered before any problematic symptoms actually arose. Even though it was a new treatment, it was considered safe for long-term use, and a 'wonder drug' panacea against the 'dreaded menopause'. The general belief was that, with HRT, unpleasant symptoms such as hot flushes and erratic bleeds could be circumvented altogether – which on the surface seemed like a good idea.

HRT involves taking prescription-only pharmaceutical drugs made from synthetic and animal-derived hormones. This temporarily prevents the natural menopause – and therefore any unpleasant symptoms – from occurring. Many people are under the impression that when a woman has a course of HRT, menopausal changes will be somehow, almost magically, taking place in the background, and that when the course finally ends, there will be no unpleasantness and the woman will be 'normal' again, only now without a menstrual cycle. Actually, though, this is not the case: menopause does not simply resolve in the background while the HRT works its 'magic'.

CASE STUDY – ELSIE

'At 85 years old, I can't believe the mess I'm in now. I've been on HRT for nearly 40 years – my doctor put me on it when I was 45, just as a matter of course as I was approaching the "change of life". It was all working fine for me, but then they stopped making the tablets I'd been taking. My doctor said they just weren't available anywhere in the world; they were an old-fashioned, high dose type. Then my trouble started! No matter what the doctor prescribed instead, no other HRT worked. My periods came back – at 85! I have hot flushes and can't sleep properly. I have become so anxious that my doctor has prescribed antidepressants, but they haven't really worked. I don't know what to do with myself!'

As you can see from Elsie's story, HRT doesn't make the menopause just disappear. At some point, your body has to go through these hormonal changes. After 40 years of being on a powerful drug, and having reached an advanced age, you would have thought that Elsie's body would have given up, and that her periods would have been ancient history. But clearly not. We have seen many other examples of cases where women, to their surprise, have suffered horrible symptoms after stopping HRT.

There is a transition that needs to take place between being fertile, i.e. having ovulatory cycles, and being post-menopausal, i.e. having no periods at all. This doesn't happen overnight, and it doesn't happen in the background. It is a natural process that takes time to complete and rebalance.

This chapter aims to help you prepare for the choices you will be presented with relating to HRT. It will give you a good basic understanding of what HRT entails, informed by examples of our clients' experience. More specifically, it will:

- help you to consider in advance what you feel about HRT;

- help you to weigh up the pros and cons of using HRT, both generally and in your particular situation; and

- suggest some positive alternatives if you choose to try those instead.

What is HRT?

The thinking behind HRT, or hormone replacement therapy, is that as natural oestrogen and progesterone levels decrease from time to time during this transitional phase of a woman's life, synthetic and animal-derived hormones can be used to compensate for any shortfall, avoiding unpleasant symptoms.

HRT doses can contain oestrogen and/or progesterone. The oestrogen is generally sourced from the urine of pregnant horses, while the progesterone comes in a synthetic form called progestogen.

The 1970s blanket approach of all women being given HRT for many years is now no longer recommended, due to long-term health risks. Instead, a more individual approach is advised, with regular reviews by a medical professional.

Current advice is to use the lowest effective dose for the shortest possible time. At the moment, medical guidelines suggest that taking HRT for five years is safe for most women. Experts who look at how medicines should be prescribed currently believe that any possible complications are outweighed by potential benefits – although this needs to be individually assessed at the time of prescription. For women who wish to continue taking HRT after the initial five years, the risk-to-benefit balance becomes less clear, and the potential for serious complications increases significantly.

The medical advice on the length of time for which HRT should be prescribed has fluctuated over the years, and this is likely to continue. This means you might be unable to remain on HRT for as long as you would ideally like. Another factor here is that local healthcare providers tend to have differing approaches as to whether HRT is routinely prescribed, or whether it is viewed more as a 'last resort' option, with women encouraged to find an alternative, more natural approach. An individual woman's particular life or health situation can also sometimes affect how long she is able to remain on HRT.

CASE STUDY – JULIA

'I had a full hysterectomy – complete removal of my uterus, ovaries and cervix – when I was just 35, because I was having a dreadful time with torrential bleeds. As I was so young, I was given HRT. I thought it was great. No more bleeds, and I felt fine. Result!

'Then, at age 53, I had a horrible shock. I suffered a mini stroke! As it turned out, it wasn't a huge deal. I recovered really quickly – in a day, actually – and I thought everything would just go on as before. But the doctor said it wasn't safe for me to stay on HRT anymore, because of the risk of blood clots or another stroke. I was hoping that I would be past the menopause, so I wasn't that bothered. How wrong was I? Hot flushes – wow! They were more than hot, and I was getting them all the time – day and night. I was moody, irritable, tearful, emotional – frankly, more than a bit mad!

'I just had to find another way. I did eventually discover Claire and Anne, and with natural supplements and homeopathy, became "myself" again. I wish I'd done this right at the beginning!'

It is important to realise that whether or not it is safe for a given woman to be on HRT at the time of prescription, things can change, and this must be regularly reconsidered on an individual basis. Should a health issue arise, HRT might have to be withdrawn quickly, and might no longer be a safe or viable option.

So, even if you find HRT useful initially, you might not be able to rely on it in the longer term.

Don't put all your eggs in one HRT basket

If you feel that HRT is a good option for you personally, it is still important to make sure that you think through how you are going to look after yourself generally. HRT doesn't give you a 'get out of jail free card'; you still have to take care of yourself, as you haven't stopped getting older. The fountain of youth has not been delivered to your door! It is worth thinking about:

- how you look after your bones;

- how you adjust your diet and weight;

- how you adjust emotionally to becoming no longer fertile;

- how you adjust emotionally to being older (and hopefully wiser!);

- what you will do if HRT is stopped or becomes no longer an option.

CASE STUDY – LYDIA

'When my menopause started, I immediately went to the doctor and demanded HRT – I just couldn't face the thought of what might happen. I didn't feel prepared, and to be honest I simply panicked. My doctor just pretty much gave it to me – I have no idea what was in it! I hadn't really thought about different ways of dealing with this – I just wanted it to go away.

'I don't really like taking medication long-term, and looking back, I wish I hadn't panicked and had been better prepared. I didn't realise I could have tried something else first. Why does no-one talk about this? All

women go through it, but I felt like it just sneaked up on me!

'After a year, I took stock, and spoke to my doctor about stopping the HRT and using diet and herbs instead. I found things that really helped. Papaya was amazing for reducing my hot flushes – who knew!'

Lydia's experience isn't uncommon. For her, a relatively short course of HRT gave her valuable breathing space to think about the menopause and what she wanted to do to help herself adjust to the changes she was experiencing. HRT was very helpful to her in those circumstances, and the benefits certainly outweighed the potential problems at that time.

In retrospect, Lydia felt she hadn't been well-informed either about HRT, its risks and its benefits, or about alternative approaches – or even about what the menopause entailed. She had simply walked forward into this time of her life, essentially with her eyes closed. So when the inevitable changes had begun, she had just panicked and become very fearful. She had done what so many women do: gone to see her doctor to try to find something that would stop it happening.

It isn't at all unusual for women to feel frightened at the onset of menopause. It is still seen by some as unwelcome and something preferably to be 'disappeared'. Most women feel unsettled and fearful about the unknown path they will have to tread. From our experience, these are the most common worries women have:

• How bad will their symptoms be?

• Will they just begin to fall apart?

• Will they lose their looks?

• Will they lose their sexuality?

• Will they lose their place in the world?

• Will it ever stop?

Think ahead

Women are not encouraged to discuss or share their concerns.
They worry that doing so can sound self-indulgent or vain.
By the time they reach their fifties, most will have spent a
good deal of their life as the pinion in their family, stretching
their personal resources to coping with a myriad of pressures
– perhaps bringing up children, caring for elderly parents,
running a home, pursuing a career, and often balancing the
financial books. They are very much the 'copers'. Thinking about
the menopause is something that often gets put on the back
burner, when actually it should be a priority.

Take time, talk to friends, do your research, find out
what you really feel. Do you have any secret fears you might
be embarrassed to admit? (Most women actually have similar
secret fears!) Or do you just need straightforward information?
(It is important!)

If you are feeling fearful – of what will become of you as
you grow older; of how you will fit into the world of youth; or of
how you will be perceived as a menopausal woman – make sure

you read the later chapters in this book. While feeling fearful is understandable, the menopause is truly a time when a woman can rise into a new sense of power and control.

Turning to HRT can make us feel like we are being given a let-off and avoiding the inevitability of ageing – initially at least. Actually, though, we are missing out. The menopause is a physical transition, yes, but it is so much more that that. It is our journey into wisdom, power and freedom.

For some women, HRT might seem a good short-term solution. Perhaps the menopause has hit with bad symptoms and, like Lydia, you need to take a breath and think for a while. Perhaps you have job or life situation in which you have to perform to a high level under stress, and HRT offers a stopgap until you can take time for yourself to process and find different solutions. Whatever the reason, if you are considering HRT, you should do your research and be informed of what you will be putting into your body.

Be informed – types of HRT available

Combined HRT involves doses of both oestrogen and progestogen (synthetic progesterone) and is considered suitable for women who still have periods but are experiencing symptoms of menopause. It is prescribed in two ways, depending on the frequency and regularity of the periods.

Women who have at least partly regular, approximately monthly cycles might be offered daily oestrogen, with progestogen taken for the last two weeks of the cycle. This is effectively attempting to mimic a natural cycle, where oestrogen is the dominant hormone in the first half, and progesterone rises and becomes dominant in the second half; the progesterone then drops at the end of the cycle, precipitating a bleed.

Women with very irregular cycles, perhaps one period every two to three months, might be prescribed oestrogen daily with progestogen taken for about two weeks toward the end of the two to three month cycle.

Continuous HRT is given to women who have had no periods for around a year and are clearly post-menopausal, but who are experiencing symptoms or have concerns about the impact of being post-menopausal – be those concerns about bone health, or mood-swings, or anxiety or vaginal dryness. It involves doses of both oestrogen and progestogen and is taken daily.

Oestrogen-only HRT, as the name implies, involves doses of oestrogen, but no progestogen. This type of HRT is suitable only for women who have had their uterus removed (a hysterectomy); oestrogen is known to thicken the lining of the womb and can cause endometrial cancer – cancer of that lining – in women who have not had a hysterectomy.

The different forms of HRT can all be given in varying ways – tablets, skin patches, implants or gels. So, if you decide to have HRT, it is important to choose a form that suits you. Those that are absorbed trans-dermally – i.e. through the skin – release the hormones more slowly, and in our experience appear to be better tolerated than tablets. When using gels, it is important to avoid skin-to-skin transference to your partner, for instance when you are lying next to each other.

So, are there any real benefits of HRT?

Broadly speaking, once they begin HRT, many women temporarily experience feeling relatively symptom-free. In other words, they have no hot flushes and, depending on the type of HRT prescribed and their current natural cycle, they might continue bleeding, although not necessarily regularly. HRT does help reduce vaginal dryness and can help overall vaginal health.

And are there any risks to HRT?

Contraindications and risks to HRT are:

- it is not recommended for women over 60;

- it is not usually recommended to be continued for longer than five years;

- there is evidence of a potential increase in the risk of breast cancer;

- there is an increased risk of blood clots;

- it is not suitable for women with history of cancer, high blood pressure, heart problems, strokes or liver disease; careful consideration needs to be given if there is a clear family history of any of these; and the treatment is likely to be stopped if you experience any of them while taking it.

Taking HRT directly affects your natural progression from a

normal fertile cycle to a settled post-menopausal position. (This progression is described fully in Chapter One, 'Understanding the Menopause'.) Your body needs a transitional period of time in order to change how it manages and accesses its hormones. During the time of fertility, oestrogen comes from the ovaries; post-menopause, it doesn't simply disappear, it is still produced in the body, but to a lesser extent. This lesser amount is now drawn from adrenal and fat tissues. This is a process of change – you could call it a learning time – for the body. It has to happen in order for you to reach post-menopause. Taking a synthetic drug overrides and interrupts this.

For women who have disruptive, irregular and chaotic cycles before peri-menopause, the temptation to seek relief from these by taking HRT can be great. It is entirely reasonable that they would like to get some predictability to their cycles. However, irregular and erratic cycles are a sign of very disordered hormones; an issue that should be resolved and not simply hidden under a synthetic drug picture. It is these women who typically experience the most extreme problems once they come off HRT, or when it stops being effective at controlling their hormones. This is what happened to Julia in the case study above.

It is much better to take steps to balance the hormones, and thus get your proper regular cycle into good shape, before considering whether or not you wish to add HRT into the mix.

Are there any medical alternatives that I can be offered?

Women at the outset of peri-menopause are often offered, instead of or alongside HRT:

• antidepressants to cope with mood-swings;

• beta-blockers to help with hot flushes; and

• sleeping tablets to help with inability to get to or stay asleep.

Women who have been on HRT but have to come off it for some reason are also commonly offered these alternatives. However, these are quite serious drugs, with addictive or habit-forming qualities, and should not be taken lightly or without careful prior consideration. It is always better to have a natural alternative if possible; and passing through the menopause means that many of the problems should resolve in any event.

What natural alternatives to HRT are available?

Although, as in Lydia's case, HRT can afford a breathing space, it should ideally be considered just that – a breathing space, and no more. It is sensible to have a long-term plan, as things can change. HRT doesn't really provide a way of moving through the menopause, or transitioning from pre- to post-menopausal states.

There are a range of proven and effective non-drug approaches, which of course have none of the side-effects of HRT. You should aim to find what works for you, depending on your own individual symptoms and personal preferences. The common symptoms are covered more fully in separate chapters of this book, and the approaches are brought together at the end to help you to devise your own strategy. For information and advice on unusual bleeding, see Chapter Two; for hot flushes, see Chapter Four; for sleep problems, see Chapter Five; for bone health, see Chapter Six; and for vaginal dryness, see Chapter Seven. Diet also has an important part to play; see Chapter Nine.

So, what is the solution?

We are used to expecting an instant resolution of annoying symptoms, but it is important to understand fully the risks, benefits and limitations of any medication. There are a myriad of strategies that women can use to negotiate their way through and beyond the menopause – many of which can be of help alongside medication, for those who choose to use it, or as standalone approaches in their own right.

Some medication is unsuitable for certain women, and all has side-effects and risks. Most importantly, none offers a life-long solution. In considering what medication, if any, you might wish to take, it is important to ensure that you are truly informed about the choices, and that you develop other practical means of ensuring your long-term wellbeing.

Time and again we meet women who feel wholly unprepared for the onset of menopause, and uncomfortable with the connotations it has been given by the media and thus by society at large – ageing, mortality, loss of sexuality, reduced attractiveness and essentially feeling that they are becoming invisible.

It is important to remember that menopause is a normal and natural phase of each woman's life, but – as with the enormous and natural change that occurs at puberty – this does not mean it will be without its problems.

Many women experience physical, psychological and emotional challenges. For some, these are mild and transient; for others, they are complex and debilitating, undermining their ability to live a normal, fulfilling life. It is important to realise that it is not necessary to suffer. Some women have no symptoms whatsoever. Having a plan is always a good idea though – in case, like Lydia, you find that things hit you out of the blue.

So, what should I do?

It is a natural reaction to be like Lydia, and panic at the onset of menopause. Most women dread this phase in their life, and the first sign that it is beginning can make symptoms worse as anxiety hits.

- The most important thing is: don't panic! Anxiety, worry and negative preconceptions are all likely to make things worse.

- Think about how you personally feel about taking control of your health. Do you want a wholly natural approach, using homeopathy, herbs, acupuncture, diet and exercise? The fact is, you will have to pass through the hormonal transition of menopause, and HRT won't permanently stop that happening – it can, though, delay it. If having a temporary breathing space is important to you, this might be a consideration.

- In our clinic, we have seen women who have gone through life not really thinking about their physical or emotional health. The symptoms they have experienced at menopause have given them time to investigate natural approaches, become in tune with their body and achieve balance. They have taken charge of their own health and now feel in control, using alternative approaches that they can now apply across all areas of their life.

- Some women – although, admittedly, only a minority – pass through menopause without a single symptom, or with virtually none. It doesn't have to be bad – so don't expect the worst. However, if symptoms do appear, there are steps that can be taken. Not only are natural approaches effective, they can positively help your body to readjust and pass through this inevitable phase as quickly and as healthily as possible.

- Don't think of the menopause as the beginning of the end, but as the beginning of a new phase.

Summary

Don't panic and rush into HRT without thinking carefully first!

HRT uses synthetic hormones that try to mimic those in a fertile cycle. It isn't suitable for everyone, and is usually time-limited. It has both risks and benefits.

Your body still needs to pass through the menopause at some stage. This can't happen while you are taking HRT.

Other natural options are available for all of the symptoms women most commonly experience

Learning more about yourself and your body, what sort of alternative approaches work for you, and what dietary changes and supplements make you feel good, has a positive knock-on impact for control of your longer-term health.

9 **DIET AND THE MENOPAUSE**

'Now I'm older and the menopause is hitting, does this mean I can eat only millet and lentils?'

That sounds like a frightening prospect! Thankfully it isn't true. What is true is that good food and good supplements provide the foundation and therefore the building blocks for good health. Eating well and staying healthy is not just about how you feel, but is essential to ensuring that the body works correctly. This includes building the bones and muscles and helping your digestion, your immune system, your hormone levels, your blood and circulatory system, your brain and memory, and your moods. In fact, everything is underpinned by diet and the foods you eat.

Wonder diets, new fads and the food 'answer to everything' seem to hit the news on an almost weekly basis. New ideas for mixing foods of different colours or of different groups, or for adopting different eating patterns, all seem to offer the way, the truth and the light. No wonder things seem confusing and frankly annoying!

This chapter explains why it is a good idea to reassess our eating habits now that the menopause beckons (or has hit!) and aims to simplify the whole question of diet.

Why are certain foods or diets recommended for menopause?

The main reasons why women look to change or restrict their diet at this time are:

- **Weight.** Many women of menopausal age find it harder than before to maintain their preferred weight. They might be a few pounds heavier than usual, and be finding it tough to shift the excess. Previous strategies such as cutting out alcohol or spending a little more time in the gym might be no longer effective. We will explain why this is happening, and help you choose the right foods to help you.

- **Hot flushes.** Some women find that either avoiding or eating certain foods can help alleviate troublesome hot flushes. However, there is a lot of confusion here, for example over the effectiveness of taking phyto-oestrogens or soya or of avoiding whole food groups such as dairy. We look at the claims, and advise which foods have been found to be most helpful and why, so that you can be better informed to decide what works for you.

- **Bone health.** There is a lot of emphasis on high calcium intake being necessary to keep bones from crumbling. We look at this in detail in Chapter Six, 'How Do I Stop My Bones Getting Weak?', but will also tell you here what supplements and food will help.

- **Generally getting older.** Your lifetime is finite, and a greater realisation of this can sometimes strike at menopause. Generally looking after yourself is probably the best reason to get a great diet that works for you. The healthier we are now – with a good diet and exercise regime and a positive outlook – the better will be our chances of living well every day as we age.

Diet – where to start?

For a lot of people, even the word 'diet' conjures up the thought of a whole series of restrictions and 'thou shalt nots'. People so often assume that there are only two options: 'boring and healthy' and 'enjoyable and bad for you'. This is not the whole truth.

Things to consider ...

Your body is robust, and perfect eating and drinking is not required! A strong and healthy body is able to cope with a certain amount of things such as alcohol, unhealthy fats and processed foods – but not excessive quantities. The body is designed to process and eliminate substances that are not good for it. This biological process keeps us alive, should we unwittingly eat foods that are not ideal or no longer in their best condition.

So, while no-one would pretend that two glasses of wine consumed over a couple of hours in an evening is a positive boon for our health, a normal liver is able to process and eliminate that quantity of alcohol over the next couple of hours. Likewise, most people have had the unfortunate experience of food poisoning, and although it can be very unpleasant, unless it is extreme, it is generally recovered from quite quickly. When a small amount of less healthy food is balanced with some good food as well, the overall health impact is usually fine.

Nevertheless, it is important to recognise that menopause is a major life change, and so needs to be supported by good nutrition.

Part of being healthy is being happy and positive, enjoying life and not making a chore of what we think we should do. Some people can become obsessional and reductionist, cutting out complete food groups – which can actually cause further health problems and reduced wellbeing.

What can be difficult is finding the appropriate balance, in view of all the information we are bombarded with suggesting incredible benefits or incredible risks associated with particular foods – all, it seems, appearing on the same page of Google!

What is it about menopause that means my body shape changes?

CASE STUDY – FRANCIS

'Previously, if I noticed that I'd put on a couple of pounds, I would cut out having wine during the week, or eat less cheese and chocolate, and my body would respond quite quickly. Then, when I reached the menopause, suddenly that couple of pounds tended to become another couple of pounds, and it didn't seem to be shifted by that quick fix – it stayed around my tummy. Help!

'Once I understood why this was happening, I looked at myself and said, "Why am I getting cross with my body when actually it is doing the most amazing, clever thing?" I did have to be a bit more careful than before with excess sugars and alcohol, but once I got my hormones balanced it was much better. Now I am through my menopause, my weight and shape are much better, more normal. I'm about half a stone or so heavier than before, but am in such a different place now that I don't really care.'

A lot of people think that the changes in body shape that accompany the menopause are due simply to their metabolism slowing down, causing them to put weight on more easily – a natural part of ageing. However, what worries many of the women we see is that this seems to happen quite suddenly. There is indeed a metabolic element to this issue – as you become older, your metabolism does become less efficient – but this is far from the whole story.

The shift in hormones at menopause plays a very important part in the changes. Many women recall that when they were younger, the contraceptive pill caused their weight to shoot up; this demonstrates that hormones can influence body shape, weight and fat retention.

Up until the menopause, women's bodies source oestrogen from the ovaries; a very efficient, easy way for them to get this important hormone. However, as the menopause approaches and the ovaries function less effectively, the body can't get the required oestrogen so easily – it has to find another way to do it. It now sources its oestrogen from the body's fat cells. This is why, very sensibly, it decides to put down a little extra fat. The fat becomes the new source of oestrogen for the longer term, moving into post-menopause.

This small additional fat store can make losing weight more difficult during menopause. So, approaching menopause with a sensible, healthy weight is a really good way of helping to stabilise the body as it goes through these biological changes.

Study yourself to decide what diet/food plan is good for you – there are individual differences

It is worth considering individual differences. Lumping everyone together and coming up with a single set of rules is nonsensical.

For example, one person could experience headaches and tiredness unless she drinks at least three litres of water per day, plus tea and coffee, whereas another might feel nauseous and bloated if she drinks even a single glass of water at once, preferring to sip it and consume no more than a litre a day – even though conventional wisdom would suggest that the sensible choice would be to drink a lot more.

This illustrates the simple point that what is good for one person might not be good for another! Finding a balanced weight during the transition of menopause is important. The right diet for you will achieve this – it will also improve your energy, gut health, immune system and brain function.

Your diet should be individualised. A carb-free or low-carb diet really suits some individuals; low-fat suits others. Trying to be something you are not is rarely successful.

Take some time and really study how you feel after meals. Does the food you eat suit you? Consider the following:

- Do you feel bloated and/or constipated?

- Is your energy low, or do you have energy dips during the day?

- Do you feel you would like to eat something an hour after a meal but don't know what?

- Do you feel like you need a biscuit or something sweet but don't really feel hungry?

- Do you snack and then feel sluggish or unsatisfied?

If one or more of the above is the case, then it is possible that your diet doesn't suit you.

Bloating, gut pain, constipation and loose stools are all signs that food is not being broken down quickly and easily. It is probably not being absorbed and used properly by your body. This will affect your gut health and immune system.

Dips and troughs in energy can be a sign that your body is not getting enough nutrition. You might also feel you want to eat 'something', but don't really know what. This is all telling you that the food you are eating is not giving you the sustained energy your body needs.

Rather than accepting that certain foods are 'healthy' and sticking with them, carefully and honestly assess how you feel after eating them.

Food having a 'healthy' label doesn't mean it is right for you personally

Complex carbohydrates, such as brown rice, wholemeal pasta and bread, are generally considered 'healthy' food. Because they are complex, it is a slow and long process for the body to break them down. On the plus side, this means the energy release from this food is slow and even. It stops blood-sugar spikes and keeps you satisfied for longer. However, some people find that their bodies don't break these foods down very well at all. They can feel bloated after eating them, and actually hungry and unsatisfied. So, for these particular people, increasing complex carbohydrates would not be a suitable approach. They might find that they put on weight and didn't feel particularly well. They would be likely to do much better on higher levels of protein.

Take the time to reflect on how your body feels, what your energy and mood are like, and how hungry or not you feel after eating.

If you are having foods that work well for your body, you should:

- feel energetic for two to three hours after eating;

- feel satisfied after eating but ready for another meal after two to three hours;

- have relatively stable energy level and mood throughout the day;

- find that you weight is stable;

- not crave sweets and biscuits; if you have one, you enjoy it, but don't feel you have to finish the pack!;

- have no gut pains, and regular good stool.

Hot flushes – can diet help?

Surprisingly, the actual cause of hot flushes is unknown, but – as we discuss in detail in Chapter Four – they are likely to have a hormonal root, as during menopause the hormones are having to go through a chemical change in order for the body to be able to process and balance them correctly. So hot flushes are not caused by diet itself. However, women often find that they can be triggered by some foods that are known to be stimulating – such as coffee, alcohol, chocolate or spicy foods – or even, sometimes, just by any hot food or drink.

It is as if the body has a problem re-regulating its temperature, which just keeps rising as it is stimulated. It makes sense, therefore, to avoid these triggers, or at least to expect the result. Exactly what brings on a flush will not be the same for all women, so be observant and follow your body, otherwise you might find yourself unnecessarily cutting out things that you love! It will also change over the course of the menopause, so experimenting with reintroducing foods from time to time is important too.

There is some evidence that hot flushes can be alleviated by isoflavones – natural compounds that bind to oestrogen receptors in the body, helping to maintain hormonal balance. We will go into this in more detail later in the chapter, as it is true not just for hot flushes, but for all symptoms of menopause, and for general health at this time of life.

We have clients who have found ground flaxseeds very helpful. They can be added to smoothies or sprinkled on cereal.

Papaya has also proved to be very effective in reducing hot flushes, as well as being recommended for bloating and constipation.

Bone health

There is a misconception that we need lots of extra calcium at menopause, to offset the thinning of bones caused by the shift in oestrogen. Actually – as covered in detail in Chapter Six – effective absorption of key minerals, including calcium, is the most important thing. Vitamin D is necessary to enable the body to absorb calcium – the calcium and Vitamin D work together to keep the bones strong and healthy.

Vitamin D is produced mainly by the exposure of our skin to the sun. Unfortunately, many of us live and work indoors – and when we do go out in the sun, we tend to cover up with clothes or sunscreen. We can get some Vitamin D instead through diet. It is found in eggs, butter, fatty fish and liver. Some foods, known as fortified foods, have Vitamin D added to them. These include some varieties of cereals, milk and orange juice.

You should consider a good quality Vitamin D supplement. Some companies also market really good vitamin supplements specifically for bone health; these typically include Vitamin E, Vitamin K, magnesium and boron, all of which help the body to absorb calcium and increase bone density. We always recommend good-quality food-state supplements; that is, supplements that have been manufactured from foods rather than chemicals. The body can absorb and use these better. Only a few manufacturers offer these, and the label will make it clear whether or not a particular product is food-state.

Diet alone will not prevent osteoporosis – you must keep your bones strong by using them. The role of exercise is vital – again, see Chapter Six for further discussion.

General health, ageing and changes in body shape

Ageing becomes more real to some women at the onset of menopause, as the inevitable changes occur, and it can feel frightening to them due to the lack of control – this is not something they have chosen to happen.

Any change in body shape is a visual reminder of what is happening, and so can become a point of fear or concern. For many women, body size and shape are important defining factors in who they are. This doesn't necessarily mean they are totally thrilled with their body, but it is them. It is how they interact with the world; how they dress; what they wear; and, in some cases, how they 'measure up'. The realisation of ageing plus a change in body shape can feel like a double whammy of things going out of control.

When we have a problem or feel out of control, we often look for an external solution. Many women therefore seek dietary solutions to sort out any symptoms and prevent the ageing process taking hold. An immediate response can be for them to go on a crash diet, or a fad diet. Sometimes they test for 'allergies' and 'sensitivities'. Perhaps they start on a succession of different food plans. All of this is looking for answers and ways to get things back under control. None of it is actually being guided by the body. We are all individual; we have individual responses and needs. Looking for a generic solution is unlikely to provide a long-term answer.

Panicking, mad diets and forcing yourself to the gym when you hate it are not needed. Starving yourself, eating food you don't like, following liquid diets and food replacement diets are all unhealthy. Actually, this kind of approach is particularly damaging to the body at the time of menopause, as it is going through very important hormonal changes that require supportive nutrients.

It is also not good to 'surrender' to the fact that the body is going to gain a little weight, and take the view, 'I might as well eat all the cream buns in the world, as it doesn't matter now.' This is not the time to deprive the body, but it is not the time to overindulge it either. So how do we feed it properly?

Following body intelligence

It is easy to get stuck in a routine of household cooking, especially when you have had years of catering for family wants and needs. You might actually have lost sight of the things you would love to eat and cook for yourself. The onset of menopause can be an opportunity to change your cooking style or food choices. Take this as a great time to put yourself first!

The hormonal changes that occur at this time might well affect the way your body uses and processes calories and carbohydrates – so take careful note of which foods make you feel bloated or tired, or conversely which give you energy or make you feel alert and fit. These might be different from those you have eaten over the previous ten years, so expect this to be an opportunity to experiment with new recipes, new foods.

Historically, it wasn't uncommon to hear stories of pregnant women eating coal. It was discovered many years later than this wasn't as bizarre as it sounded; it turned out that the coal contained some trace minerals that were lacking in the restricted diet available at the time. Of course this wasn't ideal – having the correct diet would undoubtedly have been better – but it was an example of the body attempting to find the best solution that it could in the circumstances.

How many times have you felt a desperate need for a type of food you don't normally like, only to find out later that it contains a particular mineral or vitamin that you needed? (Again, we're not talking cream buns here!) The menopause is a time to tune in to your inner voice and take note of what it is telling you. If you crave sugar, cannot open a packet of biscuits without finishing them all, or lack appetite because you feel bloated, these are all signs that you are not eating correctly. It could be that your body is craving energy on a cellular level, meaning that it isn't getting it sufficiently from your diet.

You might need to increase your protein intake, or get your protein from a different source – for example, meat instead of nuts, or vice versa. It could be that your gut flora – the collection of microorganisms in your digestive tract – is out of balance. This is often the case when you indulge cravings for sugar or carbohydrates, so you should try cutting down on those things and instead taking a good-quality probiotic (not one of the probiotic drinks on the market, as these tend to be very sugar-heavy). Taking notice of how your body feels will lead you to what it needs.

Does your body do better on four litres of water a day or just one? How do you react to bread or wheat? How do you react to meat, fish or foods that take a while to break down? How are you on alcohol; do you feel much groggier than you used to the next day? Has any of this changed significantly as your hormones have changed, and as you have aged? Always be completely honest when considering your answers to these questions. Being honest with yourself – even if not with your friends – will enable you to find an adjustment to your diet that is right for you, and help your body to go with vitality through and beyond the major hormonal and life changes that occur at menopause.

Use this time as an opportunity to find joy in cooking and eating

CASE STUDY – NATALIE

'When I saw Claire and Anne with my problems at

menopause, they encouraged me to really look at my diet. That evening I considered the food I had eaten over the course of the day and thought, "Why did I bother with any of that?" I realised that I hadn't really enjoyed or loved any of the food I'd had that day. It was just old habits; I bought the same stuff every week at the supermarket. My food was not only boring but also making me feel fat and bloated. I hated cooking, I just wanted it out of the way, so always did the same things.

'I decided to buy a blender. It came with a book of smoothie recipes, and I worked through a different one every day. I absolutely loved it, and felt better too! I had a breakfast smoothie instead of boring cereal. I love chicken, so I made myself chicken and vegetables for lunch, and loved it. Sometimes I would have a big dinner and a supper in the evening, but sometimes I realised I didn't want very much at all, and just had a salad. I no longer put things on my plate that I didn't like. My weight dropped and stabilised, and my energy levels went up. I could tell things were much better. Although my hot flushes needed more work, I knew I was on the right track.'

CASE STUDY – AMY

'I had never felt that good on rice and grains – even brown rice and wholemeal – but had stuck with them because I thought they were healthy. Then, though, I tried the Paleo Diet, which had pages and pages of ideas about

salads. Because I work from home, I often let food go cold, so having a delicious salad (not just rabbit food) next to me on the desk while I worked was really great! I made a different one every couple of days and just grazed on it, then had a meal in the evening. After a couple of weeks, I had some pasta round at a friend's house, and unlike in the past, it didn't upset my digestion. Occasionally I have bread and rice, but certainly not every day, and now my body seems to be fine with that. I don't bloat and feel "blah" like I used to. I am not strict with the diet but realise that just tending to eat this way makes me feel good. I've also lost half a stone without trying!'

Conscious eating

Many people don't really realise what they are eating, or how much. This was demonstrated in a recent television programme called Secret Eaters. The participants could not understand why they were putting on weight – they really thought there was something wrong with them. Cameras were set up in their homes, and detectives followed them over a period of time, tracking everything they ate. The participants were completely aware that they were being closely monitored, and yet were still taken aback by the findings. One discovered that he had been eating chocolate every evening; another that he had had a takeaway after going to the pub, even though he had already had a large dinner. Many were just constantly picking up and snacking on readily-to-hand things such as sultanas, crisps, biscuits and sweets.

Overall, the participants' calorie intake was measured as being between four and ten times higher than indicated by the food diary they had been asked to keep – a task they had all thought they were carrying out accurately, knowing that they were being monitored. The complete lack of awareness of what they had really eaten meant they hadn't even enjoyed it! It was a sobering lesson.

Being honest with yourself, and fully conscious of what you are eating, is important.

Your relationship with food

In our clinic we often see people who have a very poor relationship with food, and a poor self-image. This sometimes follows many years of 'unsuccessful' dieting and controlling of food.

CASE STUDY – KAREN

Karen came to see us for hormonal problems, but it quickly became clear that there were deeper issues going back to her childhood. She used food as a comfort and then, when she put on weight, decided there was no point in 'depriving' herself of the cakes she was drawn to – because it 'didn't make any difference'. In one session she confessed to standing outside a coffee shop in the rain and 'stuffing' two pastries down in very quick succession while sheltering there, before walking on down the street. She didn't even remember the taste of the pastries or enjoy them.

After we explored this with her, including in a hypnotherapy session, the core reason for her holding on to weight and turning to food for comfort and self-punishment became apparent, and we could clear that away. She was then able to become fully conscious of her eating habits, and choose food that she found genuinely enjoyable. She found she didn't need to 'avoid' cakes or chocolate, she just didn't really want them anymore. She told us, 'The sweets from Christmas are just sitting in a bowl. Normally I would have eaten them all and felt a bit sick. Now, I have one or two if I want them, but I know when I've had enough. I enjoy them, then stop.'

Karen is losing about 2lb a month steadily and happily – and feeling no anxiety about her weight or shape anymore.

The natural changes in the way the body holds fat at and around menopause can often bring out deeper negative feelings about yourself. Underlying problems can become evident. Panicking and going on more fad diets isn't the answer; in fact, with the important biological changes taking place at this time, such approaches are even less likely to be helpful than in the past.

This is a time to take stock. It is important to find what works for you, what makes you happy and what you enjoy, and to explore whether or not there are any deeper problems. You should take time to care about and value yourself, for what and who you are – and not just how you measure up physically in society.

So, I'm honest, conscious and self-reflective about the food I eat – is that it?

Many books have been written on the subject of the right diet to adopt for menopause. Some of them contain some good ideas. We will set out here the principles and ideas that have, in our experience, proved consistently helpful for most people.

The diet industry recognises that people hate being restricted in their food choices, and it has spent billions developing and tempting us with 'sugar-free' and 'fat-free' treats. Companies offer us sugar-replacement or low-calorie versions of the things we like to eat. They try to convince us that in this way we can have enjoyable and healthy food without any guilt. But, as explained below, sugar-free and fat-free alternatives are in fact unhealthy and should be avoided. We need to find enjoyable and healthy foods another way.

The following recommendations should help you to navigate your way through this maze:

INCREASE

- **Fresh food.** When your body is busy processing menopausal hormones, it finds it more difficult to cope with processed food.

- **Green, leafy vegetables.** These are very cleansing and alkaline, and have good mineral content.

- **Fresh fruits.** These have good vitamin content, including high levels of Vitamin C, and are high in antioxidants.

- **Good proteins.** These are useful for insulin and slow-release energy. Pulses are an excellent source.

- **Alkali-forming foods.** Good examples of these are nuts, seeds and green vegetables. An online search will give you a lot of other suggestions.

DECREASE

- **Red meats – especially non-organic.** These require lengthy digestion and can contain hormones.

- **Fruit juices.** These are very high in sugars, cause rapid spikes in insulin levels and affect other hormones.

- **Acidic foods – tomatoes, sweet peppers, etc.** These are especially a concern if there is a family history of inflammatory diseases such as arthritis.

- **Sugars.** These are discussed in detail below. In short, your body becomes far less tolerant of sugars than before. Do everything you can to reduce your intake dramatically.

AVOID

- **All artificial sweeteners, including aspartame and saccharin.** These cause insulin spikes and are implicated in people developing Type 2 diabetes. So, avoid diet drinks. Consider stevia products instead, if you want to replace sugars.

- **Diet/low-calorie/low-fat foods.** These often have lots of hidden artificial ingredients like emulsifiers, sweeteners etc, which are not easy to process and can affect natural insulin and hormone levels. Low-fat foods also often contain high amounts of sugar to compensate for a lack of taste and thickness.

The truth about how sugar affects you – especially at menopause

Sugar has become the new villain – sadly, for good reason. It is highly addictive, and is particularly disruptive at a time of hormonal change, because of its influence on the hormonal system.

The craving for sugar is more than just a fancy or a strong desire. It has been shown to cause reactions in the brain that are similar to those produced by taking recreational drugs. As bad as it is generally, it is even worse around the time of menopause. This is because it:

- exacerbates weight gain;

- disrupts hormone levels;

- causes mood-swings;

- causes unwelcome physical symptoms, including headaches, bloating and skin problems;

- can lead to increased incidents of cystitis and other urinary tract infections.

Another harmful aspect of sugar is the impact it has on the body's fine balance of insulin, oestrogen, testosterone and fat levels. During menopause, oestrogen is already in a very variable state; there will be days when it is very high and days when it is very low, and the body will be using the adrenal system, fat cells and ovaries to try to ride its way through the natural hormonal shifts that occur at this time. To break it down, sugar requires insulin, which is directly related to oestrogen and testosterone levels in women. It therefore disrupts the hormonal balance, and has a major impact on the changing and developing picture. This can result in prolonged and more extreme symptoms, as the body struggles to achieve an equilibrium. Sugar effectively puts your body on a mad rollercoaster, when it is already on a bit of a ride.

Like alcohol, sugar also has a stimulant effect that can exacerbate hot flushes, so cutting back on it can help with those too.

Sugars that occur naturally in foods such as fruit and vegetables (such as carrots, onions and potatoes) come as part of a whole food, and are better than other types. When the body breaks down whole foods, the sugars are slowly and correctly absorbed, so there are no unnatural spikes in their blood levels. We do need some sugars, and eating them as part of whole foods gives us easily enough to allow the body's systems to work correctly.

Concentrated foods or those with added sugars (such as fruit juices) create a massive sugar hit to the body, forcing it to make a very rapid insulin response. The insulin produced is unable to break down all of the sugar, as there is too much arriving too quickly, and instead it turns to fat. Laying down excess fat, especially at this time of life when it is harder to shift, has long-term adverse health implications. Fat can collect around the organs and the arteries, with highly detrimental consequences.

Positive food choices

As mentioned in Chapter Six, a typical western European diet is very acid-forming. Keeping the body balanced with alkali-forming foods helps the bones to stay strong and the immune system to function effectively, reducing the risk of inflammatory diseases such as arthritis, inflammatory bowel disease (IBS), ulcers and sinusitis. Simply changing the balance of your diet can be extremely beneficial, and have the added bonus of helping you to maintain a healthy weight. Your diet doesn't have to be perfect – but one or two changes can make a difference. See what works for you.

ACID-FORMING FOODS (REDUCE INTAKE)

Red meat

Dairy products

Alcohol

Wheat

Poultry

Potatoes

White rice

Pasta

Sugar

Peanuts

ALKALI-FORMING FOODS (INCREASE INTAKE)

Green, leafy vegetables

Quinoa

Almonds

Almond milk

Avocado

Beetroot

Buckwheat

Seeds and sprouts

Coconut

Flax oil

Garlic

Ginger

Pulses

Sweet potatoes

Phyto-oestrogens

As discussed in Chapter Six, there is some evidence that phyto-oestrogens can be beneficial to menopausal women. They are commonly thought of as being found in all forms of soya and tofu. However, simply increasing the intake of products such as soya milk and soya yogurts can have adverse effects, because these require a great deal of processing to make and can affect the assimilation of natural minerals, protein digestion, and natural hormone levels. A far healthier source of phyto-oestrogens is fermented soya products. There are a wide variety of these available. Try some of them out, and include in your diet those that work for you.

FERMENTED SOYA PRODUCTS

Miso

Fermented tofu

Natto

Fermented bean-paste

Soy sauce

Tamari

Tempeh

OTHER GOOD SOURCES OF PHTO-OESTROGENS

Flax

Miso

Hummus

Dried apricots/dates/prunes

Almonds/cashews/pistachios

Mung bean sprouts/alfalfa sprouts

Squash/beans/broccoli

Rye bread

Glycaemic index

The glycaemic index (GI) of a food indicates its impact on your sugar levels. Foods with a low glycaemic index have a low impact, and therefore a low impact on hormone levels too. You should aim for a 60/40 split of low/high GI foods.

LOW GI FOODS

Apples/pears

Pulses

Wholegrain bread

Oats

Mushrooms

Courgettes

Green beans

Broccoli/cauliflower

Squash

Sweetcorn/peas

Quinoa/millet

MEDIUM GI FOODS

Sweet potatoes

Berry fruits

Carrots

Parsnips

Onions

HIGH GI FOODS

Potatoes

Bananas

White bread

White rice

Sugar

Processed foods

Summary

Be honest with yourself about your diet. How do particular foods affect your energy and your mood? How do you feel after eating them?

Be conscious of what you are eating, and find the right balance for you.

View the menopause as a time of change, giving you the opportunity to try new and exciting ways of eating foods you love; new menus; new routines.

Try to make healthy adjustments and choices, keeping your life fun and food joyful.

Don't get hung up on body-shape changes – enjoy this transition, enjoy your food.

In general, a good diet at this time is one that is very low in trans-fats and meat, especially red meat, and high in green, leafy vegetables and fruit. Oils should be high-quality cold pressed types such as Olive oil and Coconut oil.

Carbohydrates influence our sugar and insulin levels, so it is a good idea to make sure these make up a small part of our diet and are not a main staple. It is easy to fall into an unhealthy habit of having toast for breakfast, sandwiches for lunch and pasta for dinner. Try to limit carbohydrate intake to one meal a day to help your hormone levels.

Processed food is not really great for anyone, but this is particularly so during the menopause, as your tolerance to it is much reduced. This can be a good time to consider a dietary supplement, both for your overall health and specifically for your bone health.

Maintaining a healthy weight is very important.

10 WAKING UP AND SMELLING THE COFFEE

The opportunities are now ...

Most of what women typically read or hear about the menopause focuses on what they will lose. They are told that their body will stop working and that they will become sexually unattractive, lose their sex drive, suffer horrible symptoms and be rendered effectively invisible. There is a lot of negative talk about the inevitability of embarrassing and unpleasant hot flushes, mood-swings, anxiety, crabbiness etc.

Actually, none of these things is inevitable. You have choices. You don't have to buy the story of lack, loss and less; it isn't the only option available.

When you think back to the first seismic hormonal transition in your life, at puberty, you will probably recall that it involved three types of changes: first, the actual physical and hormonal changes; secondly, changes in the way other people viewed you, as you moved from girl to woman; and thirdly, changes in the way you viewed other people.

The transition that awaits you now, from pre- to post-menopause, is at least as significant. It also involves hormonal changes, this time from regular fertile cycles to the ending of them. This in turn has the effect of changing your outlook and attitudes: the way you view the world, your family, your responsibilities and your relationships.

Society will accord you a changed status, too; and unlike at puberty, when it was effectively a promotion, this time it could see you being treated as of lesser worth. However, you don't have to accept this negative characterisation of your momentous and exciting change. The hormonal shift at menopause gives us more clarity, and we can see where we want to go and what really matters to us. We can decide what place we would like to take in society.

You don't have to accept the limitations and restrictions of society, or even of those around you. You can now define your own place, and your own relationships to others and to the world at large. This is the time to wake up and smell the coffee!

The fear of change

Change itself can be a frightening prospect for a lot of people. Even those who generally quite like change don't always like change they haven't chosen, and menopause is the worst kind – an enforced change!

At the beginning of the menopause, women often try, very understandably, to hold on to what they had, the past and its familiarity, because there isn't any positive discussion of 'stepping toward', or of the benefits the next phase of their life could bring.

CASE STUDY – SUSAN

'I just want something that stops this happening! My periods are going skew-whiff and I think I've had my first hot flush. I'm terrified. I suddenly feel like I'm going to

get old. I don't want to be identified as one of those dodgy people in the denture adverts, or get life cover with a free pen! How did I get here so fast? I've no idea – I just know I don't want this to happen. I haven't told my husband. I don't want any more children, but I don't want to lose the option, although I know that doesn't really make sense. I don't know what the next bit is, but I do know I'm scared about it.'

This rather panicked response to the onset of menopause is not untypical. In fact, many women would completely identify with Susan's feelings. Menopause is a uniquely challenging life change, in that women generally don't know what to expect, or what it will mean for them. All they will have heard, probably, are scary and unflattering stories. Menopause is largely portrayed as the run up to the end of life.

Rather than becoming panicked, you can choose to take this opportunity to reflect on your relationship with change. Do you love it? Or is it something that unsettles you? Imagine yourself moving house – a common type of change that most people will have experienced in their lifetime, and will generally have entered into willingly. Even if you choose and like your new home, are you someone who takes a long time before you feel it is yours? Or are you someone who relishes being in a new environment, and forgets your previous life almost immediately on moving in? Most of us are somewhere in between.

Identifying in advance of the menopause how you deal with change can be really useful. If you think you might be someone who takes time to accommodate changes in your life, then it would be worth preparing yourself, so that you can appreciate this transition and live it in the moment rather than become fearful or stuck.

Relaxing into change will really help you to enjoy this time. There are some simple things that might help

- **Bush Flower Remedies.** Bottlebrush is specifically used to help with transitions and changes. Calm and Clear combination is also useful.

- **Bach Flower Remedies.** Walnut and Rescue Remedy can be very effective.

- **Homeopathy.** Calc Carb is a remedy that helps with change generally. Ars Album or Gelsemium will also support you if you find change scary.

The transformation from woman to wisdom

The menopause is not simply a change; it is a transformation into a potentially amazing, creative and powerful part of your life. Any end of an era, or beginning of a new phase, affords an opportunity for reflection, so what is unique about this one?

There is a lot that is extremely freeing about the menopause and the hormonal shifts that it brings. Before the menopause, it can be hard to recognise the pivotal role that hormones play in controlling your life. It's not just that they can cause you a little bit of PMT (or a lot of PMT!) and leave you feeling a little weepy or angry. Actually, the effect they have on your body and mind during your reproductive years is very profound indeed.

During your fertile years, oestrogen is the hormone that influences egg maturation and ovulation. It is particularly influential in the first half of your cycle. Apart from its physiological role, it also has an important influence on your emotions and behaviour.

Essentially it is a 'make nice' hormone. That is to say, it is a hormone that helps drive your libido (sex drive), and promotes being conciliatory and caring, thus aiding the important biological reproductive role. Together with other hormones, it helps to encourage mothering behaviour, compromise and maintaining harmony by putting yourself second; in other words, sacrificing your own needs so as to care for others, such as children, partners, elderly parents, co-workers – the list goes on.

There is a reason you have had this drive. It has been important and useful. Now, though, the era has changed, and you are ready to blossom into the rest of your life.

Each human being is unique, full of possibilities. We are born with a blueprint of our future potential. During the early stages of our life, we explore aspects of this potential, first as a child, then as a young woman. But we are limited by our hormonal drives. After menopause, the power of the hormones to shape our behaviour and choices is lessened hugely.

Post-menopause, you can explore this important new phase as being your authentic self. The blueprint was always there, but it wasn't fully evident before. So it is a new time of discovery of who you really are.

Exciting or what!

Freedom, being your authentic self, allowing yourself to be

truly creative and powerful; these are things that are not dependent on external circumstances or limited by your age.

It is a time to think, 'What is possible now ...?'

Has anything been holding you back? Perhaps life circumstances and habits such as a job you hate, a relationship that isn't fulfilling, or just familiar routines of caring for a house and family. This might be a time when re-evaluation of your life becomes natural, because your changing hormones are helping you to return to your natural self, and what you truly are.

Hormones have been skewing your behaviours and choices, but now they are levelling out. This is the time for your real self to shine through. It is the beginning of the time of your life.

Finding your power, your inner you, unlocks the path to finding your wisdom. Wisdom in this sense is not about the acquisition of factual knowledge, it is about the acquisition and implementation of an insight into who you are. This is the time of growing older, yes – but much more importantly it is the time of growing into your wisdom.

Finding the real you requires that you become familiar with your instinctual energy; that is, with what you instinctively are drawn to be, what you instinctively like, what you instinctively are. You need to allow yourself to grow and develop, experiment, perhaps make mistakes, and follow a pull toward the future with joy and expectation. You can become wise in yourself and in self-development.

This is the time of growing into your wisdom with no hormones, less life baggage, and less societal expectation. For some, this involves 'growing old disgracefully', having fun and not caring what people think. For others, it might involve becoming very humanitarian, committing to charitable and giving work. For most it will be somewhere in between.

This is the essence of the complete freedom that menopause can offer. As you re-evaluate your life and future, free of the hormonal drive to cater for the needs of others, you can feel liberated. Freedom from having to achieve and fit in, freedom from caring how you seem to other people, and simply being who you are, is really the start of the most exciting time of your life. Yes, you might have a few more wrinkles, but honestly, if you try to hold back the tide of this new phase you will really be only setting yourself up for disappointment and loss.

What is this 'discovering who I am'? It all sounds a bit hippie to me!

Finding the true you means tapping back into the instinctual energy of who you are. Although there are many routes you can follow, from the conventional to the more unusual or even outlandish, one way of checking out how you perceive yourself is to do this quick quiz.

How would you describe yourself? Would you use words or sentences that denote what you do or your relationship to others? Examples are:

- I am a mother (or daughter, or sister etc – a relation to someone else).

- I am a teacher (or solicitor, or shop assistant etc – a job or a career).

- I am 50 years old (a woman of a certain age).

- I am British (or Australian, or Indian etc – of a particular nationality or from a certain region).

- I am blonde (or grey, or tall, or short etc – a visual description of what you look like).

- I am well-educated with a degree (or have a Rolls Royce, own a house etc – I have acquired material goods).

And the list goes on. All of these things are attributes (how we look or are) or acquisitions (what we have gained or achieved). None of them really captures who we are; they are just labels.

This is known in psychology as the distinction between the 'I' and the 'me'. The 'I' is just a list of characteristics and relationships to others. It is not who we really are. Can you describe yourself without starting the sentence 'I am a ….'? This can be really tricky.

The 'me', by contrast, is a psychological description of what we are; the seed, the core, that bit that is absolutely and truly us. We know that we have a body made up of cells, organs, bones etc. We know too that we have a brain that registers thoughts and enables our body to work. But there is also a sense of self that is more than these things. In other words, people have a sense of consciousness, a sense of being, a sense of self that is more than the sum of the parts of the body and the brain.

Some call this the 'higher self', some call it the 'life force' or 'consciousness', some with a more spiritual mind-set might call it the 'soul energy'. However it is labelled, this perception is something that is recognised not just by individuals, but by psychology and philosophy too.

The Swiss psychiatrist and psychotherapist Carl Jung went so far to suggest that there is a 'collective unconscious'; a shared human life energy that helps to describe and explain social and political movements.

Identifying the 'me' means looking within yourself to find your power. As this becomes your focus, you will find the 'I' energy slipping away. That you are blonde or grey-haired will become a lot less important than discovering what you love to be.

You might still prefer to have your hair dyed, but somehow the pressure to gain the approval of others or to conform to society's expectations is no longer there. If you were a child who loved to dress up and have nice clothes, this might still be part of your 'me'. If you were a child who found that all a bit boring, you are more likely to spend minimal time and effort on it. This is just the shell of what you are doing or looking like. Taking your power isn't about being the same as, or being different from, anyone else. It isn't about conforming, or conversely becoming a hippie, it is about becoming truly and authentically yourself.

The route you take to achieve this might not be straightforward, obvious or 'roses round the door'. In the discovery phase, you might have to face difficult feelings and circumstances in order that you can find out what is truly real and important to you.

What if I experience negative emotions at this time?

We cannot emphasise enough that it is okay to find this transition difficult. It is a momentous one. When in our clinic we see women who are having problems coming to terms with how they feel about their emotions at the menopause, we encourage them to explore their feelings and not to label them as negative or unhelpful.

We do see some women who come to us feeling depressed or very 'flat' at this time of their life. This can be due to emotional blocks or unresolved conflicts that they have previously scooted around – sometimes unconsciously, sometimes deliberately. Perhaps they have been able simply to ignore the issues in the past, because life has been busy. Now, though, they need to examine and resolve them.

CASE STUDY – ELEANOR

'I feel like I don't even know myself. I have a lovely husband, who keeps telling me that I look fab, but I can't even undress in front of him. I hate my body. Sex is frankly just a chore. I feel a bit lost. The kids are older now, and although I run around after them, they don't need me like they used to. I feel a bit pointless. I have always been busy, but I don't know what happens next. I've no money worries really, a good family, nice home, but things feel empty. And I feel self-indulgent to be moaning about this.'

Feelings such as Eleanor's are not uncommon, and they certainly don't make the menopause sound like a joyful and wonderful transformation. But sadly stories like this really feed the myth that it is the beginning of the end.

///

CASE STUDY – ELEANOR (FOLLOW-UP)

In Eleanor's case, we traced the negative feelings she had about her body back to her childhood, when she had felt fat and isolated, especially among her friends at school. She had never had a good relationship with her body, and during her reproductive years had had sex only sporadically, mostly when prompted by surges in hormones around the time of ovulation. We treated Eleanor with therapy and homeopathy (using the remedies Lac Humanum and Nat Mur), and she responded very well. She gained a stronger, more positive sense of her self and her body, and felt able to let go and enjoy sex with her husband. She also began to look more broadly at her life, deciding to open a new business designing textile bags, which had been her passion when she was much younger, before responsibilities had intervened.

///

When women reach the menopause, this can act as a catalyst for revealing underlying feelings and long-held weaknesses. Menopause isn't causing these; it is just bringing them to the surface. This isn't to say that emotional mood-swings aren't a symptom of menopause; however, these physiological responses can be successfully balanced using some of the self-help means described throughout this book. The hormonal swings at menopause can also shine a light on cracks that have hitherto been hidden, and allow for a more natural response to irritations and annoyances.

CASE STUDY – ANGELA

Angela was 57, and had passed through her menopause five years earlier. She had had a few hot flushes, but nothing to write home about, and thought this was done and dusted. Following recent business and money problems, her husband was now running a new business with his son, and was at last bringing in a good income. They had downsized their house and looked forward to a new life in the country, which would allow them to spend more quality time together. However, Angela felt stressed. Her family kept telling her she ought to be grateful for the opportunities she now had, and yet she wasn't happy, and was suffering lots of aches and pains.

Talking through her feelings, Angela realised that she was resentful and bitter about her stepchildren. For 25 years she had been caring for them, and hadn't enjoyed it. Her husband still babied the children, even though they were in their thirties, and her dreams and ambitions were constantly put on hold for the sake of making them happy.

She wasn't allowed to complain; her husband always reminded her that his business was paying for her lifestyle.

During her consultation with us, Angela became aware how angry she was. Up until a few years earlier she had felt okay about her situation. Recently, however, that had changed. She was no longer prepared to keep putting off living her dream for 'another couple of years'.

Homeopathic remedies helped the hormonal surges

of anger and resentment to settle, and Angela became calm and clear about her future life. She still loved her husband, but truly felt that it was not her responsibility to keep his grown-up children happy. She would be there, but would not pander to them or hang around for her husband indefinitely if he wasn't prepared to cut the apron strings.

Angela had always been this person, but during her more fertile years had felt more content supporting and making the family work, although the relationship with her stepchildren had always been a difficult one. Because she had had few physical symptoms at menopause, she had never been made aware that there could be emotional shifts too. She felt down and flat, and had been prescribed antidepressants by her doctor. In reality, she wasn't clinically depressed at all; she simply wanted her life ambitions to become a reality.

Once she realised there was nothing wrong, and that this was simply who she really was, she felt lighter, stronger and complete. She was able to let go of her anger, her whole body relaxed, and her aches and pains disappeared completely.

What do you love about your life? What really matters to you?

Being conscious of what you love about your life, what your dreams and ambitions are, and who is tempering them and why, is important. You might have been happy with your lifestyle in the past, or at least okay with it, but that doesn't necessarily mean you always will be. The subtle shift in hormonal balances that occurs during the menopause transition often means that another, deeper part of you is knocking on the door, waiting to emerge.

Finding yourself might, for instance, involve:

• Moving to the countryside.

• Sailing round the world.

• Learning to paint/dance/go crazy!

Noticing and fulfilling what you truly want right now, with no-one telling you what you 'need' to do, is the key. You will not be in a place to be told, only in a place to discover your inner self.

Hormonal changes around menopause mean we can recognise and prioritise what really matters to us – no more 'make nice' oestrogen from the ovaries, inclining us to cater for others' needs, often at our own expense. It is time to grasp acceptance of our own emotional needs.

In life, only two things are certain: death and taxes!

Without getting deep and dark about this much-avoided subject, our western mind-set is not to think about the end of our life, but to backpedal vigorously in a vain attempt to remain ever-youthful.

The menopause can be difficult to come to terms with,

because it is patently a milestone, an irreversible end to an era – and not simply a reproductive era. It means you are joining a new 'club'. The one you used to belong to, for women of approximately 18 to 49 years old, was typified by youth, fitness, career and/or motherhood, positive societal regard and respect, and a sense of material and emotional aspiration. The new one, for women of approximately 50 years old and up, might seem to have as its only aspiration the avoidance of a future of declining health, medication, stair-lifts and generally getting old, saggy and dying!

In fact, though, the passing from one era to another can have the benefit of bringing focus and clarity to your outlook. If you have been making do, compromising, waiting for the right time, this change can give you the opportunity to re-evaluate and redirect your life. You can now actually perceive the truth you have always known: that your time on the planet is limited. It becomes starkly obvious that to waste any more of the limited time you have left would be foolish.

This is similar to the epiphany often experienced by an individual who is diagnosed with terminal cancer. Once they have overcome the initial shock and grief, they will typically begin living their life absolutely to the utmost. We saw one such client in our clinic. She said she had never realised how beautiful it was simply to sit on her balcony in the sunshine, feeling the warmth on her skin and appreciating the seemingly infinite shades of green, brown and yellow of the nearby trees. Once your focus shifts to a finite length of time, it can be quite amazing how you put the trite, the boring, the unimportant and the inconsequential things to one side to make room for what really matters. There is a wonderful quote from the American philosopher and author Dr Wayne Dyer: 'When you change the way you look at things, the things you look at change.' Honestly, doing the vacuuming doesn't matter that much at all!

What truly makes you happy could be simply enjoying a sunrise, but it could equally be doing something that has always been your dream, such as starting a business, pursuing a hobby or going travelling, or perhaps experiencing something completely new that you have always meant to make time for, such as yoga, meditation or skydiving – if you've put it off before, now is the time to try it!

This complete re-evaluation can also include taking a lateral-thinking approach to your life. Very often, reaching this stage will have been a bit of a closed journey: school, university, job, children, debts, mortgage, relationship complications, money worries, and so on. Menopause, being such a definite shift, is the time for a rethink. In fact, we have treated women who, once their hormones have become balanced, have felt incredibly calm and powerful.

CASE STUDY – FELICITY

'Having been made bankrupt in the past, I was dreading having to keep on fighting financially. That horrible feeling of seeing an envelope on the mat and wondering if it's yet another bill. I could only see this situation going on into my sixties and seventies. But then I suddenly thought, "I don't need a three-bedroom house anymore. It is up to my children to find somewhere to live. My

youngest is leaving university this year." We sold our house and bought a one-bedroom flat. It's lovely. Perfect for us. When family come, they stay in a hotel, and we get on better for it. I don't have to do the dreaded Christmas dinner now, as our lounge is too small! For the first time in a long time, we can pay all our bills, love where we live, and have two holidays a year. I thought I would feel guilty letting down the children by selling their house, but they don't mind at all – they have moved on and love their grown-up lives. They say they had a lovely childhood, but that was then and this is now!'

Felicity still loved her children and was connected to them, but no longer had that overpowering sense of having to protect and provide for them – rather than just support them – that had previously held her trapped. Once her hormones were rebalanced, and she recognised her own power and ability to take her own decisions, she was able to connect to her children and family in a more mature way, and they in turn were able to respect her as an adult, with her own needs, rather than just a mother and a wife.

Felicity's epiphany was more than just the decision to 'downsize', it was the recognition of all the possibilities of her life being her own again. She rediscovered her ability to access her own intuition and realise what she wanted to be, wanted to do, wanted to live like, wanted to achieve – without the constraint of having to put others first, as she had quite naturally when her children were younger. Habits ingrained from many years of coping and making things right for others had left her in a place of forgetting about herself and neglecting to respect and love herself as a person.

Summary

If you aren't good with change generally, there are steps you can take to help prepare yourself to negotiate the major transition of the menopause.

The menopause involves hormonal changes that might make you realise that different opportunities are in front of you. It's a great time to re-evaluate where you want to go in your life, and what you want from it.

If you are struggling, there will be reasons. Explore these; don't ignore them or try to suppress negative emotions.

11 **BEING AMAZING**

In the previous chapter we discussed the reasons why menopause is a unique opportunity to open up the blueprint for the rest of your life and find your personal authentic self. In this chapter we suggest how you could break free and liberate yourself from any doubt, negativity and constraints under which you might have been living.

Menopause is the most important and profound journey you will make. Finally it gives you the wisdom, the awareness and the maturity you need to become fearless. You can now embrace your release from the biological strictures of your fertile years, and from being a 'bit-part player' in your own life. You can now use your energy and creativity as you choose. Many women have been busy having children and caring for others and haven't previously had the opportunity to explore their own potential.

The transition that occurs during and after menopause offers the possibility of changing patterns in your life. This means growing into your wisdom and finding your power – you can now embrace the joy of a natural menopause!

Spiritual growth and new possibilities

What do we mean by spirituality? Perhaps one of way of looking at it is that it is that part of ourselves that holds who we truly are. We have a sense of self; not just our body and not just our intellect, but instead a sense that we are something more than the sum of the parts we see in the mirror.

If we close our eyes and try to locate who we are, most of us feel that our body is a part of that but that there is something more. We have thoughts in our mind, but somehow those thoughts come from somewhere deeper. We have a part that gives the thoughts a voice, a feeling that we are somehow located both outside and inside our body and our mind. There is an instinctual sense of self, a sense of consciousness, a sense of our life-force and energy.

Getting in touch with our spiritual self, and experiencing growth and development, brings a sense of discovery. This is the time to seize the day; you don't have forever.

CASE STUDY – ANITA

'When I got to be 50 I thought, "Wow, here I am – I feel amazing!" My kids are very much independent; homeopathic remedies stopped my hot flushes and some of the break-through bleeding I was getting; and I feel free! I have started salsa dancing, and really don't care that I most certainly don't have a flat stomach. I have taken the opportunity to accept a short-term work contract in Switzerland. I feel I can take risks, experience more than I did before. In fact I feel like "the real me" – the me that was hidden under bringing up kids, keeping my career flying, and being sooooo sensible. No more time for that now! It's time to grab life with both hands.'

Why is this such a definitive time of growth and change? Is it just that the kids have left home and there is more free time? Or is there something special about this new phase of life? Actually, there is something special.

Your life is finite, and now is the time for you to make your mark and take charge; the time for you to realise your aspirations and find acceptance in your spiritual self.

You can achieve proper sexual freedom, and explore what you genuinely want from your partner or acquaintance! No longer do you have the risk of becoming pregnant. You can demand what you want. This is the time to become your true sexual self, whether that be actively sexual or celibate, or anything in between!

A lot of women actually describe feeling comfortable in their own skin for the first time, and losing the crippling self-consciousness about their physical body and appearance that so many younger women suffer from. This is the time to find acceptance in your physical self.

CASE STUDY – AIMEE

'I've just lost 16 stone, and I've never felt better! This is all down to freeing myself from the man who used to occupy the other side of the bed! I've had a bit of a revelation, to be honest. My new partner is a woman. I didn't think this was me, but it seems it is! We have now been together for five years. I've no idea if it will last forever, but right now it feels like a whole new world has opened up. I can't

believe I found the courage. Somehow one day I just said what I felt, and stood up for what I knew I really needed – and hey, here I am.'

We don't all have to take up with a new partner, of whichever gender, but this illustrates the kind of potential we have at this time of life. Understanding and embracing the possibilities open to you (be they small or large) is fundamental to genuinely living this part of your life.

CASE STUDY – KIMBERLY

'I've always loved yoga but thought I was very ordinary at it. Although I was very scared about my age and ability, I tentatively joined a yoga teacher training course. I realised after a few months that I was loving it. I never thought I would be teaching, it was just a pipe dream – but actually, as the course progressed, I realised that not only was I keeping up, I was getting better than some, and learning so much. It brought a whole new perspective to the group – especially the younger people. I started teaching a few classes with older women, and found I absolutely loved it. I now run weekend retreats. Originally I would have been worried about being away from home! I've met loads of new people and feel I have a whole new life that I never envisaged.

Freedom can take many forms

At this point of our life we have a myriad of amazing experiences we have learned and grown from, and most probably have already shared with others. The freedom brought by the physiological and emotional changes around menopause, coupled with the wisdom acquired through our lives, now affords a perfect storm of possibilities.

In the same way that puberty marks the division between childhood and adulthood, so menopause marks the division between the time of striving to shape the world around us, and the time of embracing and accepting the world and its possibilities. Up until now, it has been a major challenge for us to acquire knowledge and assimilate it into our spiritual side. Menopause forces us to reconsider who we have become and who we want to be, what influence we want to have in the world and what legacy we want to leave.

Coming into the era of the crone – no, it's a good thing!

The first signs that your body might be changing, such as erratic periods, unstable temperature, reduced interest in sex or increased anxiety, can bring a profound feeling of being out of control. Things are happening that you can do nothing about. This feeling of being out of control can be made worse by the negative information happily bandied about – people warning how bad your symptoms are going to become, how awful your life will be as a 'dried up old crone'.

The initial realisation that this is happening can cause a shift from a vague background feeling of age creeping up on you, to having to confront the fact that you are entering the era of being 'a menopausal woman' or 'a woman of a certain age'. Words are very powerful, and carrying a label with such negative and patronising connotations can make you feel awful and demeaned. Be conscious of the words used around you and challenge them if they perpetuate this stereotype. It isn't okay; it isn't just banter. Don't accept the ridiculous label; it is wrong at every level.

Welcoming changes actually means welcoming a new phase of your life – the crone phase, which is also known as the goddess stage. The time of power and emergence into your true self.

This new stage is transformational. In fact, you might be surprised at how different you can feel.

CASE STUDY – ALISON

'Previously, I had always had good body confidence and felt great about myself. But when I started putting on a bit of weight, and the lines became a feature of my face, to be honest I did feel a bit lost. I lost a bit of connection to myself.

'Homeopathy was great for alleviating hot flushes at menopause, but I still felt I was missing something – I just didn't know what. I kept looking at different work opportunities; I took up painting; I tried belly dancing. It was all okay, but didn't really hit the spot.

'Then a friend invited me on a Goddess Weekend. I know – what? It turned out to be amazing. We all followed *the teacher and envisaged ourselves as particular goddesses for a whole weekend. What a revelation! I suddenly found a spiritual connection to myself. I really felt the beauty of being me. The weekend ended with us all jumping naked into an outside lake. Luckily we were just out and dressed before we were spotted – which made us laugh, as we didn't even care.'*

Alison went on a Goddess Weekend, but you don't have do that in order to connect with your spirituality.

This stage needs to be nurtured

Group identity, being with people with whom you can share these new ideas and experiences, is a great way to find positive role-models and images. A Goddess Weekend is only one of the many forms this can take. Another example is U3A (the University of the 3rd Age), an organisation for retired and semi-retired people who come together to learn, not for the sake of gaining qualifications but for the sheer joy of discovery. You should explore the options and find out for yourself what suits you. You might end up trying a few things you don't like before you find those you do, but it will be worth it in the end.

There is enormous power and camaraderie in becoming part of group of like-minded people. Sharing ambitions, fears and joys and being able to identify and connect with each other, challenge and support each other, is empowering. This might or might not be age- or gender-specific. Keep an open mind and follow your heart.

Step outside your comfort zone. You might experience challenge, but challenge can be an opportunity for growth. However, don't stick with deep-sea diving if you hate it!

Some of the many things our clients have found useful are:

- yoga and meditation;

- Open University study;

- creative writing courses;

- Buddhist retreat weekends;

- retreats abroad with yoga and dance;

- ceramic-making weekends in Spain;

- surfing;

- ballet classes; and

- road cycling.

CASE STUDY – JUDY

'My relationship with my husband has been up and down for years. He doesn't treat me nicely, and it's not really what I want. I've been caught up in the angst of "Shall I stay, or shall I go?" Looking back on it now, it feels like a lot of naval-gazing. Actually, what he is or isn't doesn't matter that much. I'm doing my own stuff now. If we agree, that's great; if not, so what! The relationship doesn't define my life now, and I can't

believe it did for so long. I don't know exactly what changed. It was sort of everything. It feels like I have a new perspective on everything; I have clarity. It feels great.'

It is this clarity, this feeling of freedom, that comes now as an awakening – if you allow it to. If you struggle against it, or fight to maintain youth at all costs, this wonderful era can be lost. You have a choice between pursuing an ultimately doomed attempt to act like a teenager and becoming a powerful woman. This is the era of the crone – an era to be enjoyed and embraced.

What can be surprising is that this is a shifting and evolving picture. We can get sold on the idea that there is a fixed picture of a menopausal woman. It is as if, once you reach this age, be it 50 or 55 or whatever, you are almost frozen in time as 'one of them'. This is far from being the case.

We continue to change and grow. It would be ridiculous to think that we stop developing, learning, changing or making use of our experiences every day of our lives. There is no age at which this expansion of who we are stops. The only person who can stop it is you, either because you choose to do so, or because you allow yourself to accept the limitations that others place upon you.

CASE STUDY – SUZANNE

'I recognised straightaway the start of the menopause, and while it was a shock initially, I made a decision that I wasn't going to buy into any of this nonsense that

I would become a useless old lady. Despite my resolve, I was surprised how quickly I felt my body begin to age. Noticing this made me feel a bit down and apprehensive, and I didn't want this fear to take hold. I decided to take charge of my physical fitness, and started yoga and meditation.

'It was fantastic! It took time at first, as I had never done anything like that before. I picked a class almost at random, and discovered it was more than just exercising and keeping flexible. I learned about chakras, and how I had an inner energy I could tap into. It has transformed my life, my whole outlook, and now I have more energy again and feel the excitement of my future opening up.'

Summary

The menopause opens up a future in which you can use all your energy and creativity as you choose.

Getting in touch with your spiritual self, and experiencing growth and development, brings a sense of discovery. This is the time to seize the day, because your lifetime is finite.

Freedom takes many forms, and there are a myriad of opportunities that you have the chance to pursue.

This is your time to fly!

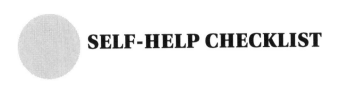

SELF-HELP CHECKLIST

The following checklist recaps the natural remedies, supplements, vitamins etc that are generally most useful for treating the main negative symptoms of menopause. Diet and exercise are also important to ensuring good health during this crucial transition period. Further details are given in the relevant chapters earlier in the book.

A good idea can be to write out your own personal action plan in a notebook or diary, focusing on the top issues that matter to you, and tailored to your own individual symptoms and circumstances.

SYMPTOM: BLEEDING

Homeopathic remedies: Sepia; Folliculinum; Carcinosin; Calc Carb.

Herbal remedies: Agnus Castus.

Topical applications: Progesterone cream; Wild Yam cream.

Vitamins (high-quality and food-state) and supplements: Multi-vitamin with high levels of Vitamins B, C, E and D; Alfalfa.

SYMPTOM: HOT FLUSHES

Homeopathic remedies: Sepia; Carcinosin; Folliculinum; Glonoinum; Amyl Nit; Sulphur.

Herbal remedies: Sage; Black Cohosh.

Vitamins (high-quality and food-state) and supplements:
Multi-vitamin with high levels of Vitamins B, C, E and D;
Flaxseed oil; Krill oil; Fish oil; Evening Primrose oil.

Topical applications: Magnesium oil.

SYMPTOM: ANXIETY

Homeopathic remedies: Carcinosin; Triple A; Gelsemium; Calc
Carb; Arsenicum Album; Nux Vomica.

Herbal remedies: Agnus Castus; Hibiscus; St John's Wort; Sage;
Menopause Support mix.

Bach Flower Remedies: Rescue Remedy; Larch; Aspen.

Bush Flower Remedies: Calm and Clear combination.

Supplements: Magnesium.

SYMPTOM: MOOD SWINGS

Homeopathic remedies: Sepia; Carcinosin; Staphysagria;
Cimicifuga.

Herbal remedies: Agnus Castus; St John's Wort.

Topical applications: Magnesium oil.

Bach Flower Remedies: Holly; Gorse.

Vitamins (high-quality and food-state) and supplements:
high-potency Vitamin B; Evening Primrose oil; Star Flower oil;
Omega 3.

SYMPTOM: SLEEP PROBLEMS

Homeopathic remedies: Passiflora; Copper Beech; Nux Vomica.

Herbal remedies: Valerian; Hops.

Bach Flower Remedies: White Chestnut.

Other: burning essential oils, e.g. lavender.

SYMPTOM: BONE HEALTH ISSUES

Vitamins (high-quality and food-state) and supplements: Calcium with Vitamin D; Vitamin E; Vitamin K; magnesium; boron.

Phyto-oestrogen sources: fermented soya; hops; dandelion; red clover; alfalfa, flaxseeds.

Other: have good exercise and good diet; reduce acid-forming foods; increase alkali-forming foods; reduce processed foods; reduce sugar intake.

SYMPTOM: VAGINAL DRYNESS

Herbal remedies: Motherwort (Leonurus Cardiac); Chaste Tree (Agnus Castus).

Topical applications: natural progesterone cream.

Vitamins (high-quality and food-state) and supplements: Vitamin C; Omega 3; magnesium.

Other: oestrogen pessaries; water-based lubricants; vaginal moisturisers; avoid perfumed products.

SYMPTOM: FEAR OF CHANGE

Homeopathic remedies: Gelsemium; Calc Carb; Arsenicum Album.

Bach Flower Remedies: Rescue Remedy; Walnut.

Bush Flower Remedies: Calm and Clear combination; Bottlebrush.

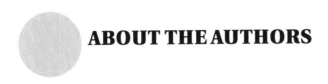

ABOUT THE AUTHORS

Claire Chaubert is an experienced professional homeopath and a qualified midwife. She lives in South East London with her family. Claire has a strong interest in issues relating to women's health and wellbeing.

Anne Hope is an experienced professional homeopath, a psychologist, a university lecturer and a yoga and meditation teacher. In 2003, she moved to the West Country, and she now divides her time running clinics in both London and Devon.

Anne and Claire trained together, and have run clinics for women in a variety of settings, including domestic violence refuges and mother and child drug rehabilitation centres, as well as specialist clinics for women's health, focusing on life development, emotional and hormonal issues, fertility and menopause. They are both registered members of the Society of Homeopaths (RSHom). They run retreats for women in beautiful settings, focusing on fertility; pregnancy; 'wise woman' workshops; and development for all stages of womanhood. This is their second book in the 'I Wish I'd Known Earlier …' series, the first being *Ten Things About Fertility That Could Change Your Life*.

Follow us on Facebook at NaturalBornHealers

www.naturalbornhealers.co.uk

Printed in Great Britain
by Amazon